about FACE

WOMEN WRITE
ABOUT WHAT THEY
SEE WHEN THEY
LOOK IN THE
MIRROR

Edited by ANNE BURT AND
CHRISTINA BAKER KLINE

SEAL PRESS

ABOUT FACE
Women Write about What They See When They Look in the Mirror

Copyright © 2008 by Anne Burt and Christina Baker Kline

Published by
Seal Press
A Member of Perseus Books Group
1700 Fourth Street
Berkeley, California 94710

Library of Congress Cataloging-in-Publication Data

About face : women write about what they see when they look in the mirror / edited by Anne Burt and Christina Baker Kline.

    p. cm.
    ISBN-13: 978-1-58005-246-7
    ISBN-10: 1-58005-246-0
    1. Self-perception in women. 2. Body image in women. 3. Women—Psychology. 4. Self psychology. 5. Beauty, Personal. I. Burt, Anne. II. Kline, Christina Baker, 1964-

    BF697.5.S43A24 2008
    306.4'613082--dc22
             2008005240

Cover design by Kimberly Glyder Design
Interior design by Domini Dragoone
Printed in the United States of America
Distributed by Publishers Group West

To our mothers,

CHRISTINA LOOPER BAKER

AND LINDA ROSE BURT,

our own first mirrors.

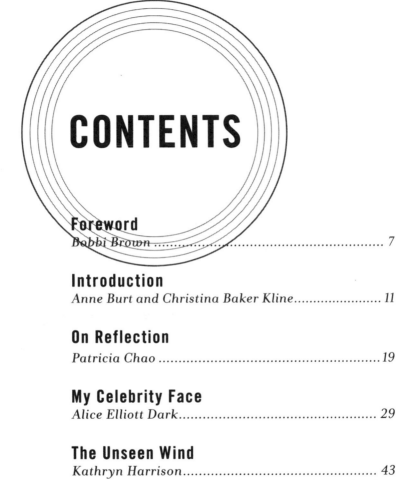

CONTENTS

bobbi brown

FOREWORD

When I was eighteen, my mother offered to buy me a nose job. I still remember the moment she sat on my bed and told me that she loved me and wanted the best for me. She said that a nose job would make me more beautiful. I looked at her and said, "You've got to be kidding." When I looked at myself in the mirror, I liked what I saw. Saying no to this procedure at a pivotal moment in my life helped me to define what I believe about myself and led me toward the work I've devoted my life to.

It's my job to hold a mirror up to women and encourage them to see what's really there, staring back at them. As a make-up artist, I want to help each woman understand, accept, and love what she sees when she looks at herself. A mirror can and should be a tool that empowers you, not an instrument of oppression. I teach the make-up artists who work for me to give a mirror to each woman they work on, so that they can see for themselves exactly how they look as the makeup is being applied.

For me, makeup has never been about hiding flaws or altering appearances; it's about enhancing what is naturally unique, and therefore beautiful, in every woman. This is the way I approach my own face when I look in the mirror and the faces of the thousands of real women and celebrities I work with every year.

This philosophy is why I think *About Face* is an important book. The writers of these essays are brave enough to talk about why their faces matter to them, and how looking—really *looking*—at themselves makes them feel. The stories are shocking and profound, humorous and poignant; they will make you gasp with recognition, nod with empathy, and laugh out loud. These writers are willing to share their deepest fears, insecurities, and secrets—feelings that all of us, regardless of our particular experiences, share.

Beauty is a lifelong journey. I've learned that it's not about looking young for your age; it's not about erasing the lines on your face; it's not about striving for unachievable perfection. Having spent my career talking to women about their faces, it's become clear to me that those of us who enjoy this journey can keep positive, stay open to growth, and learn to accept and enhance who we are at every stage in life.

I grew up in a time when beauty was epitomized by tall, blond, "all-American" models like Cheryl Tiegs and Christie Brinkley. Since I am five feet tall, with deep-set brown eyes, dark eyebrows, and brown hair, I didn't feel pretty when I compared myself with them. As I came into my own, I realized how important it is to accept the person I am and the looks I was given. In talking to women about makeup and their looks, I often feel as if I am part make-up artist and part therapist, helping women to see and appreciate the special qualities about themselves. This really isn't surprising, given that our looks are so closely tied to our identities as human beings.

The women you'll meet in *About Face* define, to me, a new "all-American" standard of beauty—one that includes a wide range of backgrounds, races, ethnicities, and ages. The youngest writer in this book is twenty-two; the oldest, seventy-five. They hail from all around the United States—some with families who emigrated from countries as far-flung as India, Mexico, Italy, and Iran. Some have learned to embrace the faces they see in the mirror; some are still actively engaged in the struggle. What they all have in common—and what they share in their essays—is that each has had a moment in her life when she realized that, for better or worse, the face she sees in the mirror defines something about who she is in the world.

Marina Budhos writes about a time when she could have chosen modeling as a career, but decided that her face would not be her fortune and chose writing instead. Kym Ragusa compares herself with a grandmother who won beauty contests and a mother who was one of the first African American magazine modeling success stories. For Ellen Papazian, it took years to wean herself from a teenage overdependence on heavy layers of makeup that literally concealed who she was. And Bonnie Friedman discovers the power of makeup only in her forties, which changes the way she now sees herself in the world.

In the end, I hope every woman will be able to look at herself in the mirror and say, as seventy-five-year-old Alix Kates

Shulman does, "We've been through a lot together, my face and I. By now we're a smoothly working team, seldom at odds, comfortable together. *Not bad*, I think when I look in the mirror. *Not bad*."

So prepare yourself to meet twenty-three women who have grappled with their definitions of a beautiful face. Reading these breathtakingly honest essays is one of the best ways to keep it simple and keep it real: Laugh and cry along with the writers in *About Face*, and you'll find a new appreciation of yourself the next time you see your own reflection in the mirror.

—*Bobbi Brown*,
　founder and CEO,
　Bobbi Brown Cosmetics

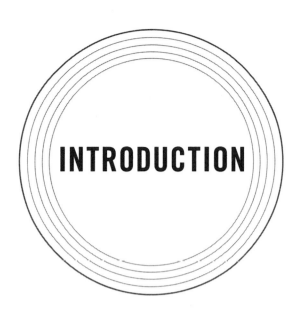

INTRODUCTION

What do you see when you look in the mirror? Those under-eye circles that have plagued you since the kids came along? A strand of wayward hair that needs to be tucked in place? When you have time to linger, is it always to fix, to coif, to pluck, to blend—or do you, every once in a while, find yourself looking into your own eyes?

Women talk about beauty all the time. We talk about frown lines and makeovers and ways to enhance our cheekbones, but we rarely talk about what we really see when we look in the mirror. What happens when we set aside our endless quest for self-improvement and come face to face with what's actually there?

You are about to meet twenty-three women who have agreed to write about the simple yet radical act of looking in the mirror. Before our society careens into a world of lunch-time liposuction and drive-thru Botox, before an à la carte menu of designer noses, teeth, chins, and eyes replaces lipstick, blush, and eyeliner in the finest department stores, we decided to step back and ask hard questions about how the way we see ourselves affects the way we live. The resulting essays reveal truths about the self in the world, and examine the societal prism through which we view, and judge, each other.

For more than three thousand years, philosophers and poets have waxed eloquent about the beauty of the female face. Girls have always grown up believing that a woman's face is her fortune, or at least her ticket to one kind of life or another.

Even today, in twenty-first-century America, deeply ingrained notions about the value and meaning of female beauty hold sway. We live in a global world, aware of many different standards of beauty. Yet the ancient belief that you can judge the content of a woman's character by the beauty of her face continues to exert a powerful influence over us. In fact, in some ways it may be more pervasive than ever.

The ancients believed that natural beauty, granted by the gods, was a mark of purity, worth slaying legions to possess. Consider the "face that launched a thousand ships," Helen of Troy. Half goddess, half mortal, Helen was so beautiful that Menelaus, king of Greece, and Paris of Sparta fought the Trojan War to win her, remaking the map of Europe in twelfth-century BCE. Then there's Xi Shi, who lived in China in the seventh to sixth centuies BCE. According to legend, Xi was so beautiful that when she washed her face in the river, fish swimming by froze and sank to the bottom. A great warrior king was so afraid of Xi's beauty that he drowned her in a lake.

Neither Xi Shi nor Helen of Troy played an active role in these dramas. Beauty itself was both their role and their fate;

their stories unfolded around them. Because the gods granted each woman her spectacular looks, even men whose lives were ruined in pursuit of this beauty succumbed to them in the end. Not for nothing did Aristotle say, "Personal beauty is a greater recommendation than any letter of reference."

But if a woman altered her face in any attempt to change the outcome of her life's events, she was reviled as a trickster, a sinner against the natural order. Perhaps the most notorious example of this is Jezebel, the biblical ninth-century BCE wife of King Ahab. Jezebel painted her eyes with kohl and purportedly committed acts of sexual immorality and duplicity. Like the sirens of Greek mythology, who lured approaching sailors with their beautiful voices, only to let them die on the rocky shore, Jezebel represents the dangers posed to men by women who employ artifice to get what they want.

Legends equating natural beauty with goodness, and artifice with deceit, still resonate with us today. In the story of Snow White, perhaps the best-known fairytale on earth, the beauty of the young princess reflects her pure heart and enrages the evil queen, whose own beauty is steeped in artifice and who shape-shifts into an ugly witch when she tries to eliminate her naturally lovely stepdaughter. As in the stories of Helen of Troy and Xi Shi, Snow White's face sends others into action, while she remains a pure, passive figure in the center. In contrast, the queen, like Jezebel, alters her face in an attempt to affect her own fate, thereby sealing her place in the popular imagination as an evil, manipulative bitch.

Our belief that we can judge the content of a woman's character by the beauty of her face is far from ancient history. There is a difference, however, between our lives today and those of older civilizations: We no longer believe that we are fated to accept the face and form we were born with—and, just as important, we now possess the technological tools to change the way we look. The very notion of fate runs counter to the principles America is built on; we are taught that with hard work, we can change anything about ourselves—finances, education, social class. Striving for a better life is not only considered admirable; it is built into the fabric of this country.

Our life expectancy is decades longer than it was when Socrates declared that "beauty is a short-lived tyranny." Women are in the public sphere far longer and for many more reasons than we were even a hundred years ago, when our sole public purpose was to emerge during our prime reproductive years to attract men and bear children. We want to look good for reasons far beyond procreation, and we have the tools at our disposal to do so. We no longer vilify women who strive to become more beautiful. But with the possibility of change comes the burden of expectation. Artifice is not only acceptable—it has become a cultural imperative.

Our contemporary mythology—delivered by movies, television, and the Internet—frames our cultural discussion and provides the kind of object lessons about beauty and character that ancient storytellers once gave us. "Tell me what you don't like about yourself," asks the fictional plastic surgeon Sean McNamara at the start of every episode of the television series *Nip/Tuck*. The only reason anyone comes to his office is to change something abhorred, something the client never wants to see when she looks at herself again. The characters in

Nip/Tuck—like "reality" television contestants and tabloid-hungry celebrities—submit to months of pain and agony to change how they look because they believe to their core that if they look better, their lives will be better. *They* will be better.

The idea that through cosmetic surgery, Pilates, self-starvation, hair dye, laser hair removal, and makeup we can attain "natural" beauty would have sent the ancient Greeks running to the mountaintops with sacrifices to the gods. But our entire beauty industry is predicated on the idea that we need not be saddled with what nature gave us. Who gets old anymore? We're too busy aging gracefully, or not aging a bit, or being only as young as we feel. Wrinkles or cellulite equals failure. Naomi Wolf, in her 1991 book *The Beauty Myth*, identified the beauty industry as a tool male society used to control women's rise in public life; yet even she fully admits that women always have and always will want to look beautiful. Our faces those we show the world, and those we show ourselves—matter.

Our goal as the editors of *About Face* is to reframe the very nature of how we talk about what we see in the mirror. We have asked the contributors to *About Face* to reveal their inner monologues that tie psychological, familial, and personal histories to the physical forms they inhabit. These writers range in age from early twenties to mid-seventies and include a multiplicity of ethnic and cultural backgrounds. Their stories tackle a range of taboo emotions: vanity, jealousy, envy, disgust.

Because self-improvement is applauded in our culture, our faces are always works in progress. We asked our writers to stop the clock and record what they see *now*. Not ten pounds from now, not Botox from now, not porcelain veneers from now, but *now*, at this moment, in all its imperfection.

This is not a book about body image, sex, or aging, though the essays touch on all of these things. We were not interested in a politically correct stance against plastic surgery; we wanted to hear intimate tales of women's relationships with their own faces. We asked contributors to go beneath the armor they present to the world and address something about their faces, their beings—and perhaps even their souls—that they might not tell even their closest friends.

About Face takes readers on a journey through the interior, into the mirrors and minds of its writers, who bravely agreed to ask and answer hard questions about how the way we see ourselves affects the way we live. Some of the questions include: What do you perceive as the relationship between your physical self and your true self? What do or don't you like about the way you look? Do you feel that your face has given or denied you access to one kind of life or another? Is your acceptance or rejection of what you see in the mirror indicative of your willingness to examine other aspects of your life? We asked each writer to include, along with her essay, a photograph of herself of her choosing.

The subjects the writers address, and the ways they address them, are as varied and nuanced as the human face itself. Kathryn Harrison turns an examination of the asymmetries in her face into a meditation on the changing nature of her sense of self, including a time when that self felt lost and she experienced a true breakdown. Patricia Chao looks at her reflection and dares to ask herself, "Who am I when I am not being loved/

seen by a man?" Catherine Texier lifts the sheet off her mother's face in the morgue and thinks, *This will be my face too when I die.* Other writers find humor in their situations, as when Alice Elliott Dark must endure hearing the man she desires comparing her, feature by feature, to the face on the Quaker Oats box. And others see a clash or a marriage of cultures played out across their very features—as half-Jewish, half-Zoroastrian Manijeh Nasrabadi finds when she rediscovers her father's roots by traveling to Teheran, donning traditional garb, and seeing her Iranian self in the mirror for the first time. *About Face* even includes essays from a mother in her fifties—Pamela Redmond Satran—and her daughter, in her twenties—Rory Satran—each examining her relationship to her face through the prism of her own generational anxieties.

It is a radical act to look in the mirror without turning away—without flinching or making excuses or posing. And it is yet another radical act to then talk about that experience honestly. Women today are no longer forced into the roles of Helen or Jezebel, but we still hold the archetypes of female beauty deep within us. Maybe what has changed since ancient times isn't the question of whether a woman's face is her fortune, but rather who is providing the answer. Long ago, we asked the gods; not so long ago, men. Now, we seek the answer from ourselves.

ON REFLECTION

Asian, long dark-brown hair streaked with henna and white, five-foot-six, slender, long-waisted, small breasted, broad shoulders, voluptuous butt, decent legs, although the thighs tend to fat. Oval face, high cheekbones, narrow close-set eyes, pixie ears, full quirky lips, nicely shaped nose. Not gorgeous, but pretty enough when I make the effort. The perfect hybrid of my Chinese peasant father and Japanese aristocrat mother. Thanks to good genes and the fact that I dress like a teenager, I can pass for ten years younger.

Tucked into the frame of the mirror I use most is a photograph taken when I was two. I am plump, with a pixie cut. My head is turned slightly to the side, and I'm sporting a smart-ass expression.

I thought this essay was going to be easy. I am, after all, a writer—trained to observe the world in general—and a dancer—

trained to observe my physical self with a dispassion bordering on coldness. And besides, what form could be more knowable than the one we view daily in the mirror? But the truth is, my reflection and I have not always seen eye to eye. And now, in middle age, there's the element of bittersweet. Or as Thomas Hardy says in his poem "I Look into My Glass":

> *But Time, to make me grieve,*
> *Part steals, lets part abide;*
> *And shakes this fragile frame at eve*
> *With throbbings of noontide.*

I still feel like I'm in my thirties. And an even more primal part of me is hardwired as a twelve-year-old—a twelve-year-old *boy*, not girl. Go figure. Maybe it's the boy in me that allows me to do this: take myself apart. Deconstruct, assess each component, separating especially the face and the body. I used to think that every woman secretly did so until I asked around and found that this was not, in fact, the case.

When I was a child, I sometimes wished for a different face. I was often the only Asian in the crowd—I grew up in the white suburbs, and my parents sent my brother and me to über-WASP private schools. I wanted to be white, or at least not so different. For many years I wished I were prettier, although when I'm honest with myself, I know I've never not gotten anything, or anyone, I wanted because of lack of looks.

But now, mostly, my face is just my face. A fact of life, distinctive, as evidenced by the baby photo I keep in the mirror. People I haven't seen since grade school recognize me instantly on the street. Lately everyone from dear friends to total strangers have remarked upon my striking resemblance to the actress Sandra Oh. I take it as a compliment. I like the way she looks—not movie-star glamorous, but very animated and human.

Still, one can dream. "You cut the suit to fit the cloth." That's my favorite line from one of my favorite movies, *The Patsy Cline Story*. Jessica Lange says it as she's examining her ruin of a face after a car accident. Women are masters at reinventing, reconstructing, improvising, fine-tuning the way we look. It takes hope, mixed with a healthy dose of pragmatism. I got a crew cut after my divorce, and later put henna in my hair, because I always secretly wanted to be a redhead. I confess to having an entire shelf of books in my apartment devoted to beauty. I don't read them much, but it's comforting to believe I could pull a Cinderella switch if I had the proper tools and techniques.

One thing I like about my face is its chameleon quality (come to think of it, Sandra Oh has this too), reflecting my chameleon nature. I am a natural traveler, blessed with the knack of blending into practically any environment. When I was growing up, friends would say: "I forget you're Oriental, you seem so completely American." But on our trips to Japan, my mother would panic because I'd disappear into the masses on the street. "You look so much like them." She never had that problem with my brother, who maintained his stolidly American persona. I once lived and worked in China for a year. After a couple of months, when I'd learned to put my hair in braids and had clothes made by a local tailor, the guards at the American embassy barred me from entering, because I looked so dissimilar to the photograph in my passport. In Brazil, where I've spent a lot of time, they think I'm Japanese Brazilian. Even on my recent vacation to Oaxaca, people started asking me if I was half Mexican. Of course, there are some places, like certain country clubs, where I can't blend in, but I at least manage not to stand out too much, perhaps because of my white suburban upbringing.

They're not mutually exclusive, but they require different heads: the ability to shine by beautifying, and the ability to become part of the tribe. The woman in me likes the former; the writer in me, the latter, because camouflaged, I can spy.

These are benign transformations. Some mirror games I've played are more serious, even dangerous. In my late teens and early twenties I battled anorexia, was even hospitalized for it. I live with the ghost. My fight to keep slender has become so ingrained in my character that I cannot imagine or remember being any other way. It's as if my life depends on it. If I'd spent half that psychic energy on writing, I'd be famous, or at least rich.

Take the years away, and you have a little girl who watches herself, in the mirror and out, with the keen, bordering-on-cruel eye of the never-satisfied parent. On the outside I was good, studious, and neat. On the inside I was chaotic, full of erotic longing. In grade school, I'd lie in bed and tell myself when I was tall enough for my toes to touch the footboard, I'd get to have sex. But I was an ugly duckling all through adolescence, shy with boys, hiding behind glasses and long hair, eating prodigiously, even for a teenager. My family doctor told me to lose ten pounds. I didn't think I was overweight, so I ignored him.

But the summer I turned eighteen, I lost my baby fat without trying, cut my hair, and got contact lenses. I invested in a wardrobe of tight sweaters—in those days, I wore a bra as infrequently as possible—and by freshman week at college, I was the kind of girl guys checked out. How heady was that first taste of feminine power! The first night at orientation, I picked out the cutest guy in the freshman class and decided I was going to lose my virginity with him by Thanksgiving—which I did, with the help of tequila and a little pot. And so it began, the insatiable hunger. From the start, for me, anorexia and body image in general have been inextricably bound up with sex. When I'm thin, I get the boys; when I'm fat, I don't. In my universe, that's been the simple, cruel truth. *Sex at all cost.* Or the subtext: *Love at all cost.*

J. Alfred Prufrock measured out his life in coffee spoons. I've measured mine in lovers, with one husband in the mix. "Why you?" a friend asked once in a drunken moment. "You're not that pretty, your body isn't spectacular, but you always have someone." It has to do with need. The only time I perfectly love my physical self—when the parts become a whole—is when I am having, or have just had, sex. Sex for me is the confirmation that I am a woman, a human being, that I in fact exist. Although I was not blessed with a va-va-voom body, I've always believed that sex is my strong suit. The little girl in the bed knew. Anorexia notwithstanding, I have always preferred my naked reflection to my clothed one. I can look in the mirror after making love and say to myself, *Yes, this is what I was made for* in a way I can with nothing else. But there's more, I know. Perhaps I need the confirmation of another human being looking at me intimately to love myself. Perhaps a man is my ultimate mirror.

Later on in my freshman year, I hooked up with my first real boyfriend, a devastatingly handsome pre-med student who played bass in a rock band. "You are just so beautiful," he'd tell me. I didn't believe him. It all felt like watching a movie. The truth was, I couldn't handle my new persona. Aside from my frenetic partying, I was spending too much time alone, much of it studying my physical and psychic reflection. The more I looked in the mirror, the more attention I got. The more attention I got, the colder I felt. I went from slender to skinny. The only thing I could think about was that finally my legs were thin enough to see the tendon by the knee. One day I saw that I looked like a skeleton. Biafra, my brother nicknamed me. But I couldn't stop myself.

Anorexia makes you want to turn yourself into a razor, an exquisitely attenuated form that shows up like a brushstroke against the background of the world. You want to be starkly seen. The paradox is that at the same time you want to disappear, lose your physical being. The line between substance and ethereality becomes blurred.

In the hospital they put me on an eating plan, and I gained weight. But it wasn't until a couple of years later, back in college as an undergraduate, that I finally felt the world again. I published my first poem, "Still Life by M. C. Escher." It's about being obsessed with one's own reflection.

I'm afraid.
Seeing is to hold to the
two-dimensional boundary,
to be contained in print.
But to be made of crystal
is to be too fragile; to only see
is to be too perfect.

I was ready to turn away from that particular mirror in which I had been drowning. But it didn't mean the game was over.

The men—an edited, annotated list: There was my boyfriend in China—a much older German painter who taught me everything I would ever need to know about eroticism and desire and tenderness and love. He bought me presents and meals—in short, spoiled me rotten—and *saw* me far more deeply than the boys in college had. I was too young to realize how rare this was. There was my husband—an absentminded, brilliant entrepreneur who turned out to be a bully. During the marriage, I became an obsessive clotheshorse, a little eighties doll. Like anorexia, it gave me the illusion of control over chaos. There was the journalist, who saw me through my grad school years, who loved me more than I loved myself; with him, I hardly ever looked in the mirror. I left him for another painter, with whom I had an on-again, off-again affair for years. Then I started dancing mambo, and that became my primary relationship, although I certainly continued with the men.

No one loves a mirror more than a dancer. You assess your body—the lines, muscles, proportions—as tool and medium, with all its possibilities and limitations. You watch yourself at rest; you watch yourself in motion. "That move looks good on you" is a common compliment dancers give each other, as if a particular step or arm decoration were a pair of shoes or a scarf, flattering to the physical self.

Mambo—as we call the syncopated street version of salsa we do in New York City—is notorious for its addictive quality. I started taking lessons as a hobby after I sold my first novel, and I fell into it heart, soul, and body—two or three classes a week, clubbing as many nights as I could manage. I knew early on I'd never be as good as I wanted, but this only spurred me on to study more, watch more, try more. Men's moves often looked better on me than women's, and I accepted this—it was that twelve-year-old boy coming out. You can't hide from yourself in dance (or in any art form, for that matter). The classic body for mambo is far curvier than the norm of beauty in white society, and my prominent butt, which I'd been dressing to diminish all my life, turned out to be a plus. On the other hand, for the first time ever, I seriously mourned my lack of tits, even considered getting implants. In salsa you need something to shake.

But inspired by the Latinas on the floor, who proudly and cunningly showed off what they had, my dance outfits became sexier and sexier, stopping just short of slutty. For the first time, I understood why men dressed in drag. I loved the exaggeration, the risk.

During the decade I danced the mambo, I was never still. My love for all things Latin took me to Cuba, and then to Brazil and Spain and Mexico, where I morphed each time into that country's version of me. My closets in New York now bristled with tropical frocks, Brazilian beachwear, Algerian lounging outfits, serapes. I even began wearing a silver cross around my neck. I dated several of my mambo partners, had a lover or two in every country I visited. All that time, I was writing furiously, a novel about Latin dance. You could call it a particularly intense middle-age crisis. You could call it coming into my own. Whatever it was, it was irresistible and all-consuming.

Perhaps it was the loss of momentum from having sold

my book, perhaps it was the waning of hormones, perhaps it was because of a particularly nasty breakup, perhaps it was because my father had a stroke and I felt my own mortality—but as I came to the end of my forties, I stopped. Stopped dancing, stopped traveling, stopped dating. I had a kind of breakdown. Occasionally I'd get dressed and made up to go dancing, but when I saw my reflection in the mirror of the lobby in my apartment building, I'd turn around and go back upstairs. I looked ugly, closed, tortured.

About a year ago, when I finally began to feel better, I met a man I decided wasn't The One, but who I knew would heal me. We were together for nine months, and it was a tempestuous ride, but there was one thing that was absolutely right: It was based on love. I'd had plenty of sex that was based on romance, as well as plenty of sex that was based on sex, but none based on love since my grad school boyfriend.

It's going to take me a while to get over this one. I have no heart to jump into another relationship. *The next one is going to be the last one* is my new motto. I have started dancing a little again—Argentine tango—although with nowhere near the fervor of my mambo days. Off the dance floor, I dress in jeans and baggy shirts and clogs. My sexual desire has been damped to a faint glow. It occurs to me that I am grieving for my youth as much as anything else. I am not in breakdown mode, but I am profoundly different from the person I was two years ago.

Who am I when I am not being loved/seen by a man? When I'm not queen of the dance floor? An extroverted stranger in a strange land? I don't know, and that's the truth of it. The good schoolgirl from so long ago tells me that I don't need to be sexy anymore. I don't even need to be thin. *Stop looking in the glass and write your next novel.*

It hasn't been easy. But there are surprises. On a recent morning after a therapy session during which I wept copiously, I came home and looked in the mirror and saw a face of astonishing beauty, somewhat ravaged by time and grief and sleeplessness, but intact and alive. I noticed a new line between my eyes, more graying at the temples. I saw the strength of my mother, the vulnerability of my niece Victoria. I saw the writer, the dancer, the sexy *chica*, the chameleon traveler. I saw the impish expression of the chubby toddler. I saw how I've tried to deconstruct my reflection, but it keeps putting itself back together.

One thing I know for certain: It will change. There is more to learn. Aging is a variation on a theme. The song continues.

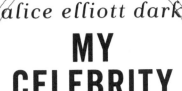

alice elliott dark
MY CELEBRITY FACE

1.

It's 1974. I'm in college. I'm in love.

At long last, after months of staring at Winston in class, I've received an invitation to his apartment. We're sitting on the sofa, trading info.

"You look like someone," Winston says. He is sitting close to me, kissably close, looking in my face.

I'm excited. He's really, really noticing me! "Who?" There's a manic edge to my voice. I'm glad he doesn't know me well enough to register it.

He pulls back. "I'm not sure. Someone famous."

"Someone famous . . . you mean, like a movie star?"

"Hmm. I'm not sure, actually."

When I was little, my grandfather said I looked like Elizabeth Taylor. It was supposed to be a compliment, but she wasn't whom I wanted to resemble, not at all. What about Patti Boyd? I loved George Harrison as much as she did. Therefore, shouldn't I look like her? So what if she was tall, thin, and blond and I was round and freckly, with curly black hair—any serious person would spot the resemblance.

Winston looked perplexed.

"Is it . . . Patti Boyd?" I said softly.

He shook his head.

"Maybe . . . Candy Bergen?" I knew I had her mouth. Our lips were narrow, bowed on top, and attractively on the pale side.

"No, that's not it."

This wasn't as fun as it had seemed like it was going to be. Too soon to give up, though—there were plenty more gorgeous movie stars where those came from. I leaned toward him, fixing my eyes on his, thinking—*Step into my magical aura, and I'll swirl my beauty around you like Stevie Nicks swirls her sleeves. I am ready for my close-up.*

"So?" I say.

He examines my smallish green eyes, my thick black eyebrows, my forthright (i.e., wide and fleshy) nose, my cleft chin, my perfect teeth. (Braces starting at age seven, due to no chin whatsoever.)

I close my eyes, ready for the kiss. . . .

"Got it!" he squeals. And giggles.

Hmm. Could giggling be romantic? I've never heard that, but the world is full of surprises. Isn't it?

"Wait here!" He's all exclamation points now; he's excited! He scampers off to the kitchen in a way that seems a bit unpromising, though I can't explain it. I'm rather unsophisticated.

Even though he has hair down to his waist and always wears green nail polish, it isn't until months later that I discover he's gay. I hear cabinets opening and closing.

More scampering. "Close your eyes!" he calls out.

Somehow I no longer think I'm about to be kissed.

"Okay, you can open them now!"

I am looking at a face, not Winston's, a couple of inches from my own. I see a blur of red white and blue, and black. A black hat. On a cylindrical container.

I recognize it, but I'm slow to get it. *What does the Quaker Oats man have to do with my celebrity face?*

"Can you believe it?" he squeals. "It's *exactly* you!"

I slip my hands under my thighs and hurt myself a little by crushing my fingers—always a reliable distraction. Otherwise, I am blank.

He looks a little hurt, like he's paid me all this attention and how can I not appreciate his massive effort?

"Really," he says. "You do. Come on. Come look in the mirror."

I drag after him into the bathroom and peer into a dingy student-rental-apartment piece of bad glass that wouldn't flatter Catherine Deneuve, much less a Quaker Oats woman. I stare at myself. The glass rolls in murky waves. Nevertheless, I see it, I see what he means. I do indeed have a colonial, leering grin, even as I'm heartbroken and frowning. I have that nose! Yet my grandfather wouldn't lie, would he? *Would he?* I look like Elizabeth Taylor. Don't I?

Winston is pleased with himself. Unfortunately, I still have a major sneaker for him. I wish I could say go to hell, but instead I say, "I see what thee means."

2.

I'm five. Starting kindergarten. I'm not nervous, because my best friend will be there too. We've been inseparable since we were two, and now we get to spend all day together, every day. What could be better? We are so close we finish each other's sentences. We're closer than we are to our siblings. We're *twins*. Or so I believe.

I spot her when I walk into the classroom. Her face is as known to me as my own—in fact, better known. I look at her far more carefully and for way more prolonged periods than I ever look at myself. I look at her so much that I kind of believe her face *is* mine. She is the same age as me, after all, and she has many of my expressions. I copy hers too. I especially like the way she holds her lips slightly apart, as if she always has a straw between them, and the way she contracts her nostrils, which I think is what makes her lips part. I love her wide, wide eyes and her long blond hair; she's beautiful. *We're* beautiful. Kindergarten is surely our oyster!

She rushes over to me, and we whisper like always. We look around, gauging the lay of the land. Her older sister has already given us a lot of tips and pointers, but even extensive intel isn't preparation for what this is really like. This is . . . other girls. Why hadn't we considered that? We imagined the room, the books, the teacher; it would be just the teacher and us, right? But there are all these other girls here, casting glances at us.

Correction: at her.

It takes only a few days for it to become apparent how different she and I are. She's the pretty one; I'm the smart one.

When we're alone, we reassure each other that we still embody the other's charms. *You're so smart*, I tell her, and she says I'm pretty. Yet it's ruined. We're not twins. The day comes when I'm put in the advanced reading group and the teacher tells her she looks like an angel . . . so much so that she'll play the role in the Christmas pageant.

I'm a shepherd. I have to wear a mustache.

3.

It's the late seventies, I'm in my mid-twenties, I'm living in London, and because I have a big body of water between me and everything that has confused me all my life, I become miraculously, with barely any effort, really, really thin. The comfy old Oats face that I've worn all my life suddenly changes into a stark, mysterious landscape of peaks and valleys, alluring as a desert or a rolling sea. Who knew what had been lying disguised all those years beneath a few millimeters of flesh?

Then, suddenly, without my even realizing it, the dream comes true. At five-foot-nine and 127 pounds, I'm a beautiful girl! Wow, what a life! Just as I imagined, only better. Like, exponentially better. Before, I'd been young and reasonably pretty, which creates its own excitement when one is out and about—construction workers politely find it within themselves to whistle and make suggestive gestures, same as they do for every young girl. A beauty, however, attracts a whole different class of street attention. Everywhere I go, I'm stared at. Every time I go into a pub or a bar, drinks are bought for me; every time I am carrying even the smallest package, a man materializes to help me on my way. It's shocking how different this world is. I'm asked out all the time, by all different kinds of men, and as I have little experience in saying no, I end up on a lot of weird adventures. I go to swanky parties, I model, I am given free clothes, makeup, jewelry. An intense Iranian man takes me to a snazzy Bond Street jewelry shop and casually buys me a watch that costs £8,000. When I say I can't possibly accept it and threaten to give it to a busker on a Tube platform, he tells me to go ahead. And I do. I drop it into a guy's hat and keep on walking. I am a beautiful girl—there's more where that came from.

People mistake me for Jacqueline Bisset. *Alien* comes out, and I am asked for autographs by people who think I'm Sigourney Weaver. I am pulled up to the front of lines at concerts and clubs. I feel incredibly free, knowing that I am liked before I even open my mouth. I feel free enough to wear a tiny black velour bikini while sunbathing in a park near my flat.

But does it make me happy?

Yup.

4.

I am in my mid-forties and at my worst. My face has completely disappeared, the bones buried under a Vesuvian avalanche of depression-slaking calories that have hardened into a slick layer of fat. I don't look in the mirror at all and can't remember if I ever did. I can't stand to see pictures of myself and hide in the back row if I have to pose. I am not who I think of as myself. My eyes have disappeared. All I have left are the Candy Bergen lips, but they hardly matter. Now's she's called Candace, and she's older too—no longer at the top of the list of world-class beauties.

Nevertheless, I'm still compared to actresses. On good days, it's Stockard Channing, the poor man's Elizabeth Taylor.

But once, someone—a supposed *friend*—says I look distinguished, like Tyne Daley on *Cagney & Lacey*. In other words, like an elementary school principal on back-to-school night. A neutered entity draped in big clothes and authority.

Excuse me while I go consult my old college diary about how to develop anorexia/bulimia. Oh, yeah: Eat only Product 19 and icing. Make yourself throw up by tickling your epiglottis and thinking of eating whatever disgusts you most.

I can't go back there, of course. I'm a mother, and certain options are off the table; suicide, inebriation, smoking, eating disorders. It's comforting to reminisce, however. Ah, those carefree days of self-obliteration. . . .

Instead I get my hair colored and join the gym.

5.

I'm fifteen, my braces are off, I have a curvy figure, and I have my first real boyfriend. He's at boarding school and I'm at home, and separation is causing me severe pain. All I can do is write letters to David and think about David. David, David, David. My vocabulary centers on this one word. I can't sleep. At night I stay up and write poems by the light of a black candle. My favorite poet is Percy Bysshe Shelley; he gets me. At about four every morning, when I'm knackered and spent, I stare blearily in the mirror, looking for that girl whom David met on spring vacation in Florida. She was hopeful and innocent, light and laughing. I don't think I even look like her anymore. My eyes are more liquid, and there's a cloud in them that is new and older. I look sad.

My metabolism slows down from this sadness, and I begin to gain weight. This causes a disconnect in my mind. Inside, I am a sad heroine who looks like Katharine Ross or Audrey Hepburn. Outside, I am one of a jillion lovelorn teenage girls who need to buy a bigger pair of jeans.

Finally David comes to see me. I hope he doesn't notice that I'm heavier. Thank God it's winter and I can wear a heavy coat. It should do the trick. We come back to my house and sit in the basement. We make out. I *love* him!

"Why don't you take that coat off?" he asks.

"I'm cold."

"But I want to get close to you."

As a concession to his desire, I slip my shoes off. They're red flats. We walked in the snow, and I see that red dye has rubbed off on my gray stockings. I'm ashamed.

"I'm fatter," I say, figuring the jig is up. If I confess, maybe I'll be absolved.

"Why?" he asks. "Why did you do that to yourself?"

Though it doesn't make me look any smaller, I shrivel.

I never see him again.

6.

I am twelve, and my mother is taking me shoe shopping. I stare absentmindedly at the back of her smooth brown hair. Everyone says she looks like Jackie Kennedy. Everyone says my younger sister looks like Caroline Kennedy. No one has ever said I look like any Kennedy.

From the back seat of the car, I crane to see myself in the rearview.

"Would you stop being such a narcissist?" my mother scolds.

We go to a store. We end up trying on the same pair of shoes together. "You two look alike," the salesgirl says.

"No we don't. She looks like her father." My mother hands her shoes back.

"They don't fit?" the salesgirl asks.

"No," my mother says. "They're too big."

"Mine are perfect for me," I say. "I'll wear them out."

7.

I'm in my early thirties, back in the States, a tad heavier than during my London glam moment, and Elvis has made a sudden appearance—not in my sandwich, or in a glass of water, but on my face. This is unexpected. I've had a poster of Elvis for a long time—a black-and-white photograph of him as a young, clear-eyed fellow—that moves me in its complete ignorance of the dissipation to come. One day I look at it, and it occurs to me—we look alike. Is this really possible? I consult the mirror. I think I'm right, but I'm not convinced, so I go get Elvis off the kitchen wall and carry him back with me to have another look. We stand side by side: him black-and-white and very pretty in his trashy, snickery way; me still hopeful and still young looking, with mischief in my eye. I curl my lip, hood my lids. We blur together in the glassy pool. Hmm—same eyes, same chin —and *same nose*. I run to the cupboard for a carton of Quaker Oats and line us all up. It's uncanny! There's a definite through line, the Scots/English genes, from Oats to Elvis to me. Somehow this seems more exciting than Jacqueline Bisset ever was. I like looking like the King—the early King, the Kinglet, not the bloated Las Vegas pathetic creature whose brilliance was subsumed in sadness and excess. No, I resemble the King who had it all ahead of him, who had the look in his eye that I see in my own childhood photos.

An eagerness, a readiness, a welcoming.

A *Here I am, world* look.

But please—love me tender. Okay?

8.

After many years of marriage, I mention to my husband that an old college pal told me I looked like the Quaker Oats man.

"That's why I married you," he says. "To keep my cholesterol low."

Funny guy. "No, really."

"It could be worse."

That's hardly the point. Don't men know they're supposed to compare you, favorably, to a major film star? Were they raised by wolves?

"What about Elvis?" I say. "Do I look like Elvis?"

"Hard to say. Elvis didn't live to be as old as you are."

9.

It's unclear whom our baby looks like. My husband and I spend hours staring at him, but this isn't elucidating. He is very small and delicate and looks like . . . a baby. But I recognize him, don't I? Somehow?

As he grows, his antecedents become clearer. Neither of us shows up in his features directly, but he does resemble both our fathers. This lasts through childhood. He's a cute kid, but that can't last forever. When he hits adolescence, there's a fresh subject for suspense: his nose.

Whose is he going to get? So far he's gotten away with a small, freckled nub. It could go either way.

Mine is . . . well . . . as described above. Have I mentioned I had a boyfriend who called me Nixon Nose?

My husband's nose is Romanesque. He's got the tallest of Rome's seven hills smack on the bridge. We each hope our child gets the other one's nose. Neither of us has ever liked our own nose, but we like each other's.

We mention to our son that this revelation will soon occur, and he begins monitoring the middle of his face for clues as to his nasal destiny.

"Damn," he says one day. "I'm getting your nose, Mom. Look at this."

He pulls me to the mirror. As if I can't see him in front of me. But okay, whatever.

"See?" he says accusatorily. "See how it's all wide and bulbous?"

"You're gorgeous," I say. "Every girl in her right mind will love you. I'd like you if I were a girl your age."

"That's disgusting, Mom!"

"I don't mean *like* like," I say quickly. "I mean—"

But he's disappeared. And taken his horrible nose with him.

10.

I'm fifteen, it's 1968, and my best friend and I are getting ready for a party. We're leaning toward the mirror next to each other, putting on makeup. She can do mascara. I'm good at blush.

I watch her look at herself from different angles.

"You know," I say, "the way you look in person isn't the way you look in the mirror."

She keeps loading the ink onto her lashes. "What do you mean?"

"I mean your mirror face isn't your real face."

"Of course it is."

"No. You're the only one who sees you looking the way you do in the mirror."

"Let's see you," she dares.

This is stupid. Why did I bring it up? Because I thought it was *interesting*. I'm interested in interesting myself.

"It's no big deal," I say.

"Come on. Look in the mirror."

I try to be natural. Which is unnatural. But that's the point.

"You're right," she says. "You look nothing like yourself." Her tone is in the awe range at this discovery, which gratifies me. I am capable of awing her, which is one of the reasons she's my best friend.

"Who *do* I look like?" I ask.

She's gone back to her work. "Hmm," she says, but she's not giving the question much thought   not the serious thought it deserves.

"Well?" I prompt.

"I don't know. Grace Slick?"

I'll take that, unconvincing as she is. Give me a minute and I'll convince myself.

11.

"He's my height," I say to my mother about my son. "You'll be surprised."

"Does he still look like—?" She names my father-in-law.

"No, I think he looks more like me now." I'm pleased with this development.

A few days later, we arrive at her house. "Oh my god," she says when she sees him. "He looks just like Elvis!"

"I look like Elvis," I say. "He looks like me!"

She shakes her head. "No, he doesn't look like you at all."

"I look like my father. My son looks like me. *We all look like Elvis.*" I explain this in a patient but uncompromising tone, as if, by being clear and firm, I might teach her something new at this stage of her life. I am still the young, hopeful Elvis, it seems. I even look like him again. I've lost weight. No more gray hair. I've shaped up.

"No," she says. "Just him."

Her certainty inflames me. I'm regressing fast here. In seconds, I'm thirteen again. "Who *do* I look like, then? You said Candy Bergen!" I want her to *leave me alone*, but not before I have her complete approval.

"No," my mother says with great authority. "That's your sister."

"My sister? She looks like Caroline Kennedy!"

I stop. What am I talking about? My sister looked like Caroline Kennedy when she was a child.

Sometimes we have moments of grace—not Grace Kelly— when we see ourselves accurately. In my case, and in the case of a lot of women I know, this is rare. Our mirror faces are contorted to what we can tolerate. We hate photographs of ourselves because they show us what others see when they look at us—and those faces rarely match our longings.

This, however, was a bracing moment of truth. My sister, I thought, doesn't look like little Caroline Kennedy—not anymore. She is an attractive middle-aged woman with a look of her own.

As am I.

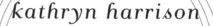

kathryn harrison
THE UNSEEN
WIND

*Nature gives you the face you
have at twenty, life shapes the
face you have at thirty, but at fifty you
get the face you deserve.*
— COCO CHANEL

*I'm twenty when my father looks at me and says, "You know,
you've never seen your real self. I have, but all you've seen is
your reflection in the mirror. An image that looks very much
like you but isn't the same as you. Not really, not exactly."*

"Why wouldn't it be exactly the same?" I ask, irritated because he's always doing this: telling me why I belong to him and
not to myself.

He explains that light is lost inside a mirror; a reflected
image lacks the luminous property of the object itself. As an
experienced photographer, he conveys authority about such

things. "Try it," he says, and he pulls me next to him before a mirror. "Look at me," he says. "Look at the real me here beside you, and then look at my reflection. They aren't the same. You'll see they aren't the same."

I don't want my father to be right. I don't want him to own what he says he does—the way I *really* look—leaving me with what he makes sound like an approximation of myself, inexact and indistinct, no better than a Xerox. But when I compare the actual man to his image, I see he's right—they aren't the same. The mirror father is dimmer, duller, not quite alive.

So it's true, what he says: I have never seen, and will never see, the real me.

The divine ratio of Phi—1:1.618—determines what nature gives us. Phi unwinds the chambers of a nautilus and the spiral of a galaxy, arranges seeds in the head of a sunflower. Phi is the principle on which Leonardo da Vinci based his illustration of a perfectly proportioned human being, arms and legs spread wide, the top of his head, the tips of his fingers, and the soles of his feet all points on a single circle. The ratio 1:1.618 is the length of the hand compared with that of the forearm, the width of the face to its length, the width of an eye to that of the mouth, of the eye's iris to the eye itself. Phi is the mathematical constant, sometimes called the Golden Ratio, exemplified in Renaissance portraits and in the portfolios of Ford models.

Symmetry. Harmony. Balance. These are beauty's terms, her demands. Exacting, like Coco Chanel. I don't fulfill them. I know this before I do the math, dividing the length of my face by its breadth, comparing the width of my mouth to that of my eye. It's too long, my face, either that or too narrow. My ears are where they ought to be, but they're too small. And while no one's features are absolutely symmetrical, I think mine may be a little more off-kilter than most. Or perhaps it's this I notice first when looking in a mirror: a lack of symmetry.

I play the old game of covering one side of my face to analyze the other. The woman I see when I cover the right side of my face, showing only my left, is approachable, engaged. She appears pensive, but not so preoccupied that a stranger would hesitate to interrupt her thoughts to ask directions, say, or inquire whether she's using the empty chair at her table. The woman I see when I expose only my right side is another story, an altogether darker character. Not sinister, but wary and untrusting, hidden deep within herself. Aloof. She must be the one I hear described as icy.

"'The ice queen'—that's what we called you when you came in for your first interview," a coworker tells me when I'm twenty-seven.

"You're kidding," I say.

"No, really. That's how you came across before we got to know you." We laugh, because in reality, I'm often the first to poke fun at myself or crack a joke in a meeting, to let down my guard in hopes that others will too. I know what he means, though. No one has ever put it to me quite so starkly, but the shock I feel when he says this to me is one of recognition.

"You have to smile at people," my husband tells me. We haven't been married long, not even a year. "You have to look people in the eye and smile at them when you meet them," he says. "Otherwise, they think you're unfriendly. I know you're uncomfortable with people you've just met, but they don't know you like I do."

Slowly—it takes ten years or more—I teach myself to be the left side of my face when in company—congenial company, anyway. Because the right-side woman does have her place, her usefulness. The right side guards her thoughts, whatever they may be, discouraging idle conversation and unwanted confidences. She isn't rude or unkind; she'd give up the unused seat at her table. But a stranger might hesitate to ask her for it. Seated next to her on a train or an airplane, other passengers don't try to draw her into a dialogue. She makes it clear she doesn't want to talk, and in this way, she guards my privacy, my space, and my time. It's she who ensures I can read my book uninterrupted.

My eyes account for the difference. The left opens wider; its brow is half a centimeter higher than the right's, enough that it alone is visible above the frames of most sunglasses, greatly reducing the number from which I can choose. Because the left eye is wider, literally more open to inspection, it appears to welcome the curiosity of strangers, while the right remains comparatively hooded, defended if not defensive.

I smile at myself in the mirror, trying to discern if the woman I see is a friendly-looking person. And I frown, as I do when I'm concentrating, to make sure the frown doesn't look ill-tempered. But what use is this? Any face I make for myself is self-conscious, artificial; it tells me nothing about how I might appear to others. Perhaps this is why I've never practiced expressions in a mirror. Even as a teenager I was sure they wouldn't be the same as the ones I would really end up making.

Although there is one trick I attempt to master. In my

twenties, entranced by a friend's ability to raise one eyebrow independently of the other—entranced by her in general, as she is very charming—I determine to teach myself her way of using one lifted brow to make a silent inquiry or convey disapproval more subtly than words allow. But I can't get the hang of it. It never appears effortless or natural. Instead, I look like our dog does when she hopes to avoid a scolding, her head cocked to one side, her forehead wrinkled in anxiety. Under the single raised brow, my eyes betray the strain of concentration; they make me a picture of vulnerability and self-consciousness, the very qualities that inspire my desire, at that age, to look superior.

"If you make a face and the wind changes, it will stick," my grandmother tells me when I am very young. I believe this— I believe everything she tells me—and I worry: What if I am inside the house and I make a face, not knowing that it's windy outside? My face could be frozen forever in a grimace, or a look of surprise, my mouth a round O that I would never be able to close. I resolve to arrange my features into a pleasantly neutral expression and keep them that way, so as to defeat the unseen wind. But no, this will never work. I can't remain conscious of what my face is doing for even a minute.

A winter morning, a Saturday. I am no longer a child but a woman of thirty, and my grandmother is ninety-one. The passage of time has reversed our roles; now I am the parent, she the child. Still, her power is such that I remember all her pronouncements: that if I were to step on a needle, it would travel through my bloodstream and pierce my heart; that if I cross my eyes, they won't uncross; that opening an umbrella inside the house or putting shoes on a table invites disastrously bad luck. I don't believe any of these, not quite, but I don't forget them either.

The two of us are readying ourselves for a trip to her hairdresser, and then on to the supermarket, where each week we walk slowly together through the long aisles and she picks among the groceries, squandering as many minutes as she can on each choice: among brands of crackers, boxes of dry cereal, patterns printed on rolls of paper towels. It's her only outing of the week, and she looks forward to it, and to having my undivided attention for as long as my patience for marketing lasts. I go downstairs to her floor of our house to see if she's dressed, and find her in the bathroom, the door left open. Still in her housecoat and slippers, she's looking at her reflection. Outside the window, snow is on the ground, and light falls on the tiled floor in long, blue-white bars. My grandmother is so small and bent that the mirrored door to the medicine cabinet can't show her any more of herself than her face, and she looks at it for some moments, holding herself straight so that her chin makes it into the mirror's frame.

She doesn't see me in the hall outside the bathroom door; she doesn't know I'm watching her. Slowly, she reaches forward over the sink and touches her reflection. "I've grown old," she says, speaking to no one. "Suddenly, I've grown so old." There's wonder in her voice, mystification: How has she failed to notice what must have been happening for some time?

It's a private moment, or I might move to comfort her. Not that I could dispute the truth she apprehends, but I might try to distract her from it. I might make tea or suggest we sit by a window where we can watch the people on the sidewalk as they pass before our house. These are among her favorite pastimes—making and drinking tea, watching strangers as they go about their business.

But it's not a moment I can enter, only one I can destroy with my intrusion. I go back up the stairs, knowing that I've seen the arrival of my grandmother's awareness of her death, its imminence. Knowing also that I won't forget what I've seen; it belongs to me as well as to my grandmother, and I will carry it forward; it will become part of my apprehension of my own mortality, a thing so certain and unavoidable and even so natural that I imagine myself standing, one of an infinite line of women, generations going forward as well as backward, from my too-many-greats-to-count grandmother to the grandmother I know, to my mother, long dead, and on to myself, to my daughter, and her daughter's daughter. As if my grandmother or I, any one of us, were caught and multiplied between opposing mirrors, I see all of us reach forward to touch this harbinger of our deaths—the face, once a maiden's, now a crone's—trying to understand what we can't understand, because how can Being grasp Nonbeing? How do we picture it, the absence of ourselves?

It's not the same as what transpires between my grandmother and her reflection, but one day I look into my bathroom mirror and find that the person I expected to see isn't there: She's disappeared. The two moments are separate, divided by years, as I am thirty-seven at this point, and my grandmother is no longer living. And yet they are connected.

I am more seriously depressed than I can admit or even perceive, only a day away from what I don't anticipate—a stay in a psychiatric hospital. Not sleeping or eating, unable to work or think straight, I've gotten into the habit of comforting myself with a photograph that reminds me who I am, who I used to be. It's a snapshot my husband took. I'm sitting with our children in a field of summer wildflowers, all of us bathed in light that looks genuinely golden, light that is a benediction, evoking chalices, redemption. We're smiling; the wind lifts my son's pale hair into a halo. I use this picture of us to call me back into myself, reorient me to what is the essence of my life. It works well, too, until suddenly it doesn't work at all.

The children are in school, my husband at work. I look at the photograph and don't recognize anyone in it. *Who are these people?* I think. *Who are they to me?* I wait for the image to take effect, to reach past whatever is wrong with me, but nothing changes. I know I'm supposed to know them, *us*, but they're no different from the people who come flattened under the glass of a newly purchased picture frame, a set of smiling strangers whose likeness you're meant to discard and replace with a picture of your own.

I put my snapshot away in the drawer, walk into the bathroom, and stand before the mirror, staring. Apparently it's possible, from one day to the next, from one hour to another, to slip out of one's skin, one's self, and land in a new, alien, and unrecognizable face.

Time passes—months, then years—and the bathroom mirror that shows me I'm not sane loses its power to frighten me. Still, I find it mysterious, and even wonderful, that there would be so stark and irrefutable—so apt—a symptom of a nervous breakdown as a failure to recognize one's own face.

My husband and I discuss a piece of art made by our older daughter, who's going off to college soon. It's a life-size self-portrait, the final project for a course in advanced drawing. I think it's quite accomplished, I tell him. Especially I like the placement of the figure in the frame, and the way she's rendered her hands, which, I point out, are difficult.

"But look," my husband says, "that's not her face. Her nose isn't that short, and her mouth doesn't look like that. And the eyes are the right size but not the right shape, not exactly." The problem is, he concludes, our daughter has fallen prey to an idea of how she looks, and this idea is different from how she really looks. She's drawn the face she believes she has, or wants to have, because that's the face she sees in the mirror—the idealized one, rather than her own. We continue to talk, about the drawing, about magazines and TV and movies, and how what media presents as beauty may influence, even create, our daughter's idea of her face. Perhaps she can't see her face as clearly as she might were she not trying to render herself in a society so eager to tell her how she's supposed to look—to define the contours of a perfect face, to direct attention to certain details over others, to make one face an icon, another unworthy of notice.

The idea stays with me long after our conversation ends. Each of us must see our physical self through a lens of various influences: prescriptive advertisements; critical remarks made by parents or lovers; the human tendency to conflate physiognomy and character, mistaking a high forehead for intelligence or full lips for sensuality. Perhaps when we are young, we're more easily enthralled by the faces of certain models or actors—affected by something beyond their looks. We assume, of course, that powers are granted them by celebrity and imagine these might belong to us if only we looked as they do. But perhaps the psychic trajectory is more complicated.

Couldn't it be that we project what we wish were true of ourselves onto the faces of famous strangers, finding heroism, self-confidence, dignity, genius—whatever qualities we aspire to possess—in the way they appear? Don't we mistake their faces for illustrations of what we desire in ourselves and then try to emulate what we see, or even begin to believe we look a little like these more nearly perfect avatars, these faces of who we might, with effort and time, become?

And wasn't this what I lost or inadvertently broke ten years earlier, when I didn't recognize myself: my idea of who I was, who I am? That lens of influences and aspirations, whatever apparatus would have guided my self-portrait: I must have lost what allowed me to bring myself into focus.

I ask my husband if he doesn't think it must be difficult, maybe impossible, for our daughter to see herself at seventeen. She has what nature has given her, but she hasn't yet lived long enough to fully inhabit those features. How can she know what she looks like when the past years have been experiments in identity, trying on personas and shedding them like the clothes strewn over her bedroom floor? At fifteen she said she would never wear Birkenstock sandals, which were "ugly, gross, stupid." At seventeen she has a pair she wears all the time. She loves them, she tells me. "You didn't used to," I remind her. She shrugs. "I know," she says, "but that was then."

My daughter's father wouldn't say to her what mine did to me, that he sees what she cannot: her real self. His greater age might make him immune to what informs her vision, but his eye must be subject to other, different forces—among them that power long equated with blindness: love. If we separated our senses from our emotions, we would be less than human. If we could see anyone for whom we have strong feelings clearly— ourselves included—we'd be far more evolved than we are; we'd be divine.

At forty-seven, do I know my features better than my child knows hers? Sometimes I'm startled by the face I see reflected back at me. Not the countenance I review each morning, unfolded from sleep, washed and subjected to quick analysis, to moisturizer, tweezers, and whatever corrections I can effect with cosmetics. Without expression, less a whole than a series of parts revealed by a magnifying mirror, that face is little more than a list of tasks to accomplish: teeth to brush and floss, brows to check for stray hairs, under-eye circles to mask with concealer, lips and lids and lashes to color. I'm speaking of a face I see inadvertently, cast back at me in a shop window as I hurry through errands. Who is that woman? Whose dark and angled glance meets my eye in a department store mirror I don't anticipate? She looks to be a solitary soul, the face who catches me unaware; she looks anxious and driven. A face I glimpse rather than see.

Actually, it must be I who catch her, for she's the one who flees—the right-hand side of my face, the one with the hooded eye, the side I thought I could banish and summon at will, using her to silence garrulous fellow travelers or defend me against the occasional boor. Apparently she isn't obedient but emerges according to her own agenda, knifing efficiently through sidewalk crowds, punctual and humorless and . . .

. . . and me. As much me as the left-hand side, with her wide, dreamy eye—the self I own more readily because she's attractive, flirtatious, quick to smile, to laugh. The lines she's traced on my face are lines I like, radiating out from each eye. Different from what the right-side woman has etched into my forehead.

Perhaps the unseen wind did change one storm-tossed day when, heedless of the consequences, I was looking as I felt: dark and brooding, overcast by fears. That face stuck, and others did as well—the one, for example, I wore when sitting in a field of wildflowers, golden.

My grandmother didn't say I'd have only one face. She didn't say it couldn't happen again and again with every shift in the wind. That was my misunderstanding.

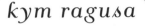

kym ragusa

THREE WOMEN, THREE PHOTOGRAPHS

MIRROR

7:00 AM: Looking into the mirror for the first time today, I see a blur. Without my glasses, which I discovered I needed just after turning forty last year, it takes my eyes a moment to focus. And then the first thing I see, as always, is my skin. My nakedness and my cover. My shelter and my vulnerability. The color of tea with milk, slightly sallow, a suggestion of rose in the cheeks. My face is wide, with broad cheekbones and a rounded half moon of a forehead. The curves of the top of my face contrast with the sharp angles of my chin and jawline. My eyes are drawn next to my hair, six sleep-fuzzed braids, the color of wet bark, twisting and curling around my cheeks and down to my collarbone. My eyes are still puffy and a little bloodshot from a night of confused and troubled dreams. They are almond-shaped, and now that I'm paying attention, they are lighter than I had thought, brown irises with a brightness behind them, ringed with black. I have long, feathery eyebrows, slightly arched, with a shadow of stubble between them where I've neglected to pluck. Below my left eyebrow is a small, raised, red birthmark, like a fairytale tear that has dried into a jewel. My nose is small and broad from the front, though long and pointy from the side, and my lips are round and pale. I've always thought that their roundness made them look like a question, and in fact my face—my features and my coloring—have always provoked questions. Why do I look like this?

MAP

I have a map of the northeastern United States, marked with red circles in the places where my various ancestors lived and died. My first known ancestor on this soil—an enslaved woman whose mother was an African, from where I don't know, and whose father was her mother's German master—was born on a plantation in Maryland. She died in Pittsburgh, Pennsylvania, the city she escaped to with an Irish man with whom she eventually had ten children. From there, the red circles fan out across the map: a Cherokee great-great-grandmother born in the Smoky Mountains of North Carolina; a red-haired, almost white great-grandfather born in the Appalachian mountains in West Virginia; another great-grandfather who came from China to work on the Western railroads and who died in Virginia, where he had opened a laundry; a grandfather who traveled in steerage from southern Italy and died in suburban New Jersey. Red circles overlapping, generations layered into the map, like layers of sediment in rock, my family's history fused into this varied and changed landscape. Red circles overlapping, a map of blood, the bloodlines crossing and meeting in me.

CONTEST

In 1951, the *Chicago Defender*, an African American newspaper, held a beauty contest and invited black women from all over the country to enter. My maternal grandmother had been a journalist, writing society columns for a number of black newspapers, and my husband, researching a project related to the newspaper, did a search for her name in its archives. What came up in the search results was not my grandmother's journalistic work, but the beauty contest, apparently an advertising ploy to get women to buy subscriptions to the paper. The caption reads, "Contestants from Coast to Coast Make Early Bid for Fabulous Prizes." Ten thousand dollars in cash for first prize. Below, along with a list of contest rules, is a row of eight photographs, each featuring a contestant, and my grandmother is one of them. Looking at this image of her now is shocking. It's not that my husband pulled it from the abyss of cyberspace, or even that she entered the contest in the first place. It's her beauty. The women in the other photographs are demure, with high necklines, upswept hair, pearls at their throats. They are all light-skinned, which is not surprising, given the ideals of beauty among many African Americans at the time. My grandmother, though, is flaunting her light skin. Unlike the other images—all head shots, like high-school-graduation or driver's-license photographs—my grandmother's is a medium shot. She's leaning against a wall, in front of what looks like a film advertisement, in a black, spaghetti-strap dress with a deep décolletage. Her lips are painted dark red, her hair falls across her eye in a Veronica Lake wave. Her expression is haughty, chin up, eyes tilted slightly downward. The extravagance of her sexuality, the extravagant lightness of her skin, makes me want to turn away in shame. By the time I was born, my grandmother had become a political activist; she spent the 1960s and '70s protesting unfair housing practices in New York. In those years she wore a curly afro and brightly colored caftans. And somewhere along the way she developed a disdain for sexuality, an aversion to physical desire. This was the grandmother I knew: a woman passionate for justice for her people but self-contained, almost reclusive, in her private life. The beauty-contest photograph feels somehow like a dirty secret unearthed. Exposure: a reaction of light on the receptive surface of paper, my grandmother's skin revealed, responsive and unguarded.

PORTRAIT

Following in my grandmother's footsteps, my mother worked as a fashion model in the 1970s and '80s. I grew up with images of her, clipped from newspapers and magazines, that my grandmother collected and kept along with her own glamour shots from the 1950s. For a while, my mother lived in Europe, strode catwalks in Paris and Milan, got bit parts in B movies shot in Rome's Cinecittà. Where my grandmother was a conventionally ideal beauty in the black communities to which she always felt she belonged, my mother was an exotic in the fashion worlds of Europe and New York. She had skin the color of raw honey and wore her hair in what seemed like thousands of tiny braids, falling down her back, rustling when she walked. She used to have a photograph of herself that hung above the fireplace in her apartment in New York. It was a portrait taken by the fashion photographer Francesco Scavullo: a close-up of her face, surrounded, I think, by white fur. She was smiling, and in the small gap between her front teeth was a heart-shaped diamond. It was an image of herself my mother loved—an idea of beauty as currency, as wealth. But like the white mink coat that hung in her closet and the diamond cross she wore around her neck, the portrait was eventually lost. Divorce, age, the omnivorous desire for the next new face in an unkind industry—my mother couldn't keep the wealth that beauty momentarily brought. And as her things disappeared, something of my mother was lost too. The memory of the portrait—dazzling, excessive—has become the memory of her, of how far she reached before she fell.

PHOTO BOOTH

When I was in my early twenties, I lived around the corner from a novelty store that had a working photo booth. It began with a random visit alone one day—I slipped into the booth and turned around just before the flash went off. Five minutes later, the strip of four photographs slipped down into the drying slot, still damp, with an acrid chemical smell. Four shots of the back of my head—I never turned to face the camera. For a year after that, I photographed the back of my head, recording the changing seasons of my identity, my femininity: from the time that I wore my hair, as now, in a few lopsided braids,

to the time I cut it short and bleached it until it glowed a sickly orange, to the time I shaved it off completely. After that, I
recorded the patterns and shadows the stubble made on the
back of my head. I had seen the photographs of Lorna Simp-
son, who shot images of black women with their backs to the
camera, and I was fascinated by that refusal of the gaze, the
refusal to play the sometimes obscene game of beauty, or lack
thereof. I knew too the history of photographic images of black
women—the anthropological studies of "Hottentot Venuses";
the portraits of enslaved women, concubines and property; the
fantastically ambivalent film stills of Josephine Baker dancing
in a miniskirt made of bananas; and the self-portraits of black
women artists who challenged these earlier representations.
I knew these images, but I don't think I was consciously ad-
dressing them in my visits to the photo booth. More immediate
in my mind were the memories of other photographs, those of
my mother and grandmother. I spent much of my life looking
at their pictures, memorizing their outfits, their poses, their
flashed smiles. I was someone who looked—being looked at
was another matter. The representations, and the living images, of my mother and grandmother were almost too much
to bear. Their beauty was dead weight—what it got them didn't
last, and they carried it alone. And I, thin, sallow, shy, couldn't
compete with their breasts, their lips, their skin. Those photo-
booth pictures were a game to me then, an art-school affecta-
tion. But I wonder now what it was that I was really refusing.
Was it the gaze of history, or of desire? Was I protesting a kind
of representational violence, or displaying my own loneliness
and insecurity? Why didn't I turn around?

MIRROR

Twenty years later, I face the mirror. And what I see is a map. My skin, my eyes, my hair: They are not beautiful, and they are not ugly. They are the traces of all the people, the women and the men, who took a chance, who left all they knew to begin again, the people who came together to make me. The people who traveled an ocean, who walked down a mountain, who crossed borders both physical and metaphorical—and risked everything. And even my grandmother, entering a beauty contest, believing she could change her life; and my mother, smiling her gap-toothed smile in anticipation of all that might have been possible, for her and for me. Whatever I believe about their choices now, I see their longing in my face. This is my self-portrait, a map of overlapping dreams and desires, of blood mixed and blood spilled. Neither ugly nor beautiful. Skin, hair, eyes, nose, mouth. It has taken me half a lifetime to account for these features, how they've combined to create my face. An accounting both public and private. Why do I look like this? Go back; go back through the family snapshots, the immigrant portraits sent back to the Old Country, the ethnographic field photographs, the antebellum daguerreotypes, the fashion shots clipped from magazines. I'm there in all of them, the kink of my hair, the tilt of my eye, the light glancing off my skin.

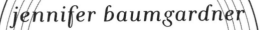

jennifer baumgardner

MS. WORLD
OF WHEELS

Dazzling, streaky-haired Gloria Steinem once said something along the lines of "No one thought I was so beautiful until I said I was a feminist," which was probably somewhat true but not the whole story. Steinem was, I think, riffing on the popular myth about feminists: that we are ugly, too grotesque to get a man—and therefore our habits of running for office, landing a seat on the Supreme Court, or writing books are merely elaborate justifications for having no date on a Friday night. Steinem was also deflecting the notion that she is more beautiful, and thus more powerful, than other women due to her big hair, great smile, cute nose, legs made for miniskirts, sylphlike bod, high cheekbones, and soulful brown eyes. In reference to Steinem's statement, Helen Gurley Brown once remarked to me, "Well, she would say that—because she's gorgeous. She doesn't know what it's like *not* to be gorgeous."

I looked at Helen—seventy-something at the time of the conversation and dressed in a sparkly minidress and perky, brand-new breasts courtesy of a surgeon—and wondered whether I was a Helen (sharp, scrappy, itching for entrance into the pretty-girl world) or a Gloria (graced with pulchritude but eager to be taken seriously).

As a child, I was definitely a Helen. I had *small* hair, for instance: It was short and androgynous, courtesy of my parents, who insisted that—with what they called my "elfin" chin and petite physique (if you overlooked my Streisand nose)—I would look best with a buzz cut.

"Can I help you, son?" shop clerks would ask during this phase of my youth.

"I'm a *girl*," I'd mutter, humiliated by their mistake.

The first time I remember feeling consistently pretty was age ten, when I finally got to grow my hair out and would create elaborate hairstyles in the bathroom before school while my five-year-old sister, Jessica, gazed at me from her perch on the toilet, enraptured. I'd part my golden locks in the middle and curl the bangs back in the 1970s fashion (though it was by then 1980, I lived in Fargo, North Dakota, where we came to styles late and held on longer). Then I'd take a hank from the front part and make a braid, finished with a clear bobbled ponytail holder. That year was the first year I was among the popular girls. Or at least not a total weirdo with a witch nose whom people mistook for a boy. I had boys looking at me; I was pals with Brita and DayNa and the other precociously lovely blonds. I had admirers—or at least I had my little sister.

I don't recall when I first considered myself a feminist,

but the philosophy was right there in my 1970s milieu, in the sneaker skates and white bikini I wore while roller-discoing to Donna Summer, as my dad pulled up in a large Oldsmobile with a SUGAR AND SPICE, WILL IT SUFFICE? sticker on the bumper. I grew up with *Ms.* magazine and a mother who gave me a copy of *To Kill a Mockingbird* when I was eleven, when she caught wind of a book report I handed in about *Valley of the Dolls.* I was born into "Free to Be!" "That Girl!" "Mary Tyler Moore!" "Maude!"—and I reflected those cultural messages. I wrote letters to the editor of the newspaper in support of abortion rights at age thirteen. My father taught me how to throw a punch without breaking my thumb. I was proud of being smart.

On the other hand, beauty loomed large in my young psyche. I wrote Brooke Shields a letter begging her to be my pen pal, and my fondest dream was to be discovered and whisked to New York City to become a model. I bought all of the fashion magazines and found *Ms.* dry. By the end of high school, I knew I *shouldn't* care how I looked, because the content of my character was much more important, but I also sensed that I was less vulnerable to being seen as a boy, lesbian, or outcast if I was also pretty. Partly because of temperament and partly due to genetics, I was never going to look like the peppy, button-nosed bouffants who made up the various cheerleading squads at my high school. So I tried to be something else: a *Dynasty*-era Joan Collins bitch. Someone who conveyed being above it all but was still gorgeous—in a mean way. I cultivated snobbishness and wore shoulder pads that Nolan Ryan would have loved.

My desire to be beautiful was rooted in my desire to be powerful. There were lots of ways to have power, but it seemed important to have "looks power" first. Life went on like that for a while. I was obsessed with my face, my mood totally transformed by a single compliment and sunk into a Nietzschean dilemma ("Do I exist?") if a construction worker failed to catcall. (And, as a teen at least, I was totally freaked out when I did get attention from men. Life was a big freakout.) But this was my secret self. My real self was being a smart snob in vintage clothes who was truly bored with these small-town inanities. Which is why I'm so surprised that I ended up in the World of Wheels pageant in 1987.

The World of Wheels was a car show, held at the civic center in Fargo, but they also had a beauty pageant called Miss World of Wheels. The prize for this competition was $500, which to my junior-year pocketbook was like what $10,000 would be today. I could use that money for college or more shaker-knit sweaters from The Limited, I thought, and I signed up to compete. Now, this was a car show—and the people attending wore trucker caps and T-shirts and had nonironic handlebar mustaches. I was, if I haven't made this clear yet, a theater geek with Morgan Fairchild aspirations. I sang songs from *Fiddler on the Roof* on weekends; I loved Liza. I had a figure like Carol Burnett (my idol) and the pale, lovely (if nauseated-seeming) visage, replete with short bobbed perm and bee-stung lips, of Molly Ringwald—my other idol. The other women—many were older, in their early twenties—in the pageant had the five Bs: bronze tans, boobs, and big, blond bangs. They wore bikinis; I donned a fashion-forward gold lamé one-piece. The minute I entered the pageant's doors, I could see I was not in a world where my sartorial daring or my other attributes (such as my ability to sing "Macavity" at full throttle, my large vocabulary, my pro-choice politics) would be valued.

My sister Jessica was in the audience and recalls having a "lamb to the slaughter" sensation when I took to the stage for the interview portion. When I was asked whether I liked to tan (seriously, that *was* the question), I—glowing with near albino paleness—decided my only chance was to default to pretending to be above these small-town, low-class grease monkeys. "No," I answered, full-on Ringwald dyspepsia inflecting my tone. "I'm sorry, but no one should tan. It causes skin cancer." Jessica said the crowd stiffened en masse and looked as if it might boo me, the buzzkill, off the stage, then thought better of it. After all, the lady who came after me had a great bod, was brown as a nut, and actually valued the "sun, cars, and alcohol" mantra of the World of Wheels.

I forgot about competing (and losing) in the World of Wheels for years. I went to college, where I actually got a great deal of attention for my looks—my high cheekbones, pretty blond hair, and tall, lithe figure. After high school, girls with brains got a better deal, and I was alive with the fresh beauty of a late bloomer. I no longer had zits (thank you, Accutane) and was actually sort of a dead ringer for Kelly Lynch in *Drugstore Cowboy*. By the end of sophomore year, I was also a rabid college feminist. First, we protested the mutilated dolls that a male artist made, learning we could be a united front of outrage and could scare people. Later, drunk on power and flat beer, we would talk at the frat parties about how women should have guns and the only good rapist was a dead rapist. We were hot bundles of tough, miniskirted contradictions.

After college, I moved to New York City, the epicenter of glamour, but also a place where people like me escaped to. If you spent your childhood in a small town, plotting revenge and singing show tunes, invariably you would find yourself in Manhattan as soon as you could. The city, like feminism, offered an exciting new value system—beauty was measured differently, your whole self was taken into account. If you were scintillating or *jolie laide* or brave or raucous or all of it, welcome to New York! I no longer felt shame about the part of me that longed to be powerful in that most basic, most perishable female way—the part of me that wanted to be beautiful. In fact, by New York standards, I seemed wholesome and sweet. Relatively speaking, I had become that perky blond cheerleader. I even modeled here—nothing big, but I was the "face" for a boutique cosmetics company, my picture in displays at Sephora stores, and I did a spread for an Italian fashion magazine, among other piddly but ego-boosting ventures.

For a long time, I couldn't talk about things like the World of Wheels pageant, or being told to lose weight at the modeling agencies I went to when I first moved to New York, without coming up with a justification for why I put myself through the gauntlet. And the rationale was (like Gloria's saying she wasn't *that* pretty) partly true, but not the whole truth. I'd say that before I became fully conscious, I engaged in tribal rituals of female debasement before the male gaze. "I would *never* do something like that now, *thank God*," I'd say. What I didn't say is this: It wasn't competing that felt so bad. It was trying and failing. Getting chosen to do the modeling for Sephora or *Moda Italia* felt great. I can admit that now. After all, feminism can't say there is no place in its philosophy for beauty or raw power. To survive, it has to be like New York—to glory in beauty, but never value a woman just by that measure.

I'm now a thirty-seven-year-old single mother of a three-year-old, and I'm feeling older by the second—from my sleep deprivation-induced Russell Crowe eye bags to my Jell-O belly to my mortgage payment-anxiety forehead wrinkles. On a good day, I resemble Aimee Mann—on a bad day, an old man. Recently, my book *Look Both Ways* was reviewed in a fashion magazine, the kind I read as a teen. In it, the writer referred to me as "by far, the hottest of the Third Wave feminists." In truth, I felt a little zing of accomplishment. I had come full circle. I was beautiful—for a feminist.

manijeh nasrabadi

SOUVENIR

Oh, so that's what I look like, I thought. It was April 11, 2004, and I was twenty-eight years old. The mirror was old, dingy, had been hung there on the back of a door in my uncle's crumbling old house in central Teheran long before I could even imagine such a house, such a man, existed. But my reflection was new. Ordinarily, I'd have done a quick, instinctive scan of each of my facial features—like checking for danger in both directions before crossing the street. That day in Teheran, though, I didn't do this. I didn't separate my face into component parts to be scrutinized or lamented. In the home of my father's brother and his family, I saw my face as one whole face for the first time.

For most of my life, Iran was a just a setting for my father's stories—less real to me than Mr. Rogers's neighborhood

---

The author has chosen to include a childhood photo to protect her identity.

of Make-Believe, which at least I could see with my own eyes on TV every week. My father was born in a place I had never seen, a small clay village outside the desert city of Yazd, where his Zoroastrian family had lived for generations. His stories drifted from village orchards and squares—replete with traveling storytellers who unfurled painted scrolls—to the euphoric street demonstrations that clogged Teheran's broad avenues and ushered in Iran's first democratic government. The excitement in my father's voice would rise, as if he were still standing among the hopeful throngs, and then crash to a bitter register when he talked of the coup that followed, the executions, his own close encounter with the secret police. In 1979, he came back from a short visit to Iran with a new set of stories about how his people had kicked out the bad guys, Iranian and American. They were going to build something called socialism, he said, and it was going to be like a dream come true.

I was five, growing up in Washington, D.C., and my life was confined to the few blocks between our house, my school, and the baby sitter's house. This story of revolution was too incongruous, unfolding on too grand a scale, for me to grasp. I did gather, after a few months, that it didn't have a happy ending, and that the whole thing seemed to only to make my father upset, something a good story should never do to its storyteller.

In the 1980s, while one million Iranian and Iraqi soldiers were battling each other to the death, my younger sister and I were children at war with our reflections. She and I had an ongoing, intermittent conversation, among the earliest I can remember between us, in which we examined the minutiae of our parents' features, pulling them apart in our minds—like the interchangeable parts of our Mr. Potato Head toy with the removable face pieces—to see which of us had gotten what. The same way in which we knew what arrangement of parts was the most normal-looking for our plastic potato, we also took for granted that my mother's facial attributes (white, European) were more favorable than my father's (brown, Iranian). Even now I hear a little bell chiming for a feature of my mother's, and an offensive buzzer sounding for one of my father's, like on some sort of twisted eugenics game show where the contestants are required to judge themselves.

After lengthy discussions, we agreed that my sister had our mother's eyebrows, thinly drawn and in no need of plucking. She also had the recessed bone structure of our mother's eyes, but she had our father's round-shaped face and chin, with a slight dimple in the center. I had our father's bushy eyebrows, which tormented me when I reached adolescence, and his large almond eyes—the only feature I actually liked. My face was the oval of our mother's, but with my father's rounder cheeks, and deemed by some (including my mother) to be exotic-looking— which always sounded to me like a euphemism for "freakish" and "pitiable." My sister and I both had our father's coloring, with skin somewhere between olive and brown. In a rare display of unity, we hated our noses. We understood from a young age that this largesse of both our Iranian and European Jewish lineages, in any combination, could be nothing but hideous. Even as a child, I felt something desperate and sickly in this self-dissection, as if I were both scientist and specimen— a strange hybrid creature who, having discovered myself, was now cataloging my various parts.

Out in the world, things became only more confusing. When I was with my Ashkenazi Jewish mother, shopping at the mall or visiting her law office, people were surprised to learn we were related, because I didn't have her blue eyes and fair skin. I could only try—through my speech, through my gestures—to show I was just as American as she was. But despite my best efforts, I heard again and again, "*That's* your daughter? You look nothing alike."

When I was with my father, whose skin is dark from the desert sun, I found his obvious foreignness embarrassing. Thrust unwillingly into the role of interpreter, translating from English to English, from one kind of accent to another, I would try to smooth out the awkward interactions he'd have with neighbors and shopkeepers along our way. Sometimes, I could tell that they were put off by the same things that secretly ashamed me (his effusive, overbearing compliments, for example, or his habit of standing so close to people that they would involuntarily back away). I found myself worrying about how they saw me.

The most troubling thing about my reflection was this: It was unreliable. The image I saw was never the one I expected to see. In the beginning, when I played with the white little girls from my elementary school (in my memory, there were only white little girls), it didn't occur to me to think about how I looked. Over and over again, I was caught off-guard by my own face. In the first grade, after school in Annabelle's blue-carpeted attic playroom bursting with toys, there was a mirror idly leaning against one of the diagonal A-frame walls. I didn't notice it until it was too late.

"You be the teacher, and I'll be the student," Annabelle said. She had light blue eyes, a button nose, and long, straight, dirty-blond hair. Her cheeks were pink, and her arms were dotted with light beige freckles, like my mother's.

"Okay." I felt lucky to get to be the teacher.

"Go down the stairs, and then when the bell rings, come in," she said.

I went about halfway down the stairs while she sat on the floor and settled into her makeshift cardboard desk, an old bicycle bell at the ready.

When I heard the bell ring, I walked up the stairs in as dignified a manner as I knew how and beamed at my pupils. "Good morning, everyone."

"Good morning, Mrs. Roberts," Annabelle said, as if in chorus with the rest of the class. Mrs. Roberts was the name of our actual first-grade teacher, whom we both loved and feared. "Now say that we're going to have a quiz," Annabelle stage-whispered.

"Okay, class. Take out a piece of paper. We're going to have a pop quiz."

Annabelle groaned, rolled her eyes and pulled a piece of paper out from a pile on the floor. There was a chalkboard against one wall, on which I was supposed to write some of the numbers we'd learned to add. Chalk in hand, I passed by the mirror on my way. Something caught my eye. *That's* what I look like? My nose was enormous, pointy, and hooked like something that ought to be covered up. Paralyzed for an instant, I forced myself to keep walking, to stand with my back to the make-believe class and write addition problems on the board. But that face haunted me; it didn't add up with the way I felt on the inside. *That* was what pretty little Annabelle saw each time she looked at me? I didn't want to play our game anymore, even if I was the teacher. I wanted to go home and hide in my closet on the bottom shelf that was just wide enough for me to sit on, almost invisible in the near-darkness.

Back at home, when I stood alone in front of the mirror that rested on top of my dresser, I sometimes thought maybe I looked okay. Maybe what I saw in that other mirror was a mistake. Maybe when people looked at me, what they saw wasn't really so bad. But I couldn't be sure.

I fought against this loss of control by keeping a vigilant watch, stealing glances in car windows, in glass storefronts, and in the small mirror I came to carry with me always, a shameful concession to my preoccupation that I tried to peek at as clandestinely as possible. I couldn't decide which was worse, not looking and imagining my face undergoing a sort of reverse chameleon effect, morphing to become more obviously out of place; or the humiliation I felt when I did confront the mirror and despised what I saw. A Muppet. A monster. Since I had no words for this peculiar form of torment, I couldn't explain it to my parents or my sister, and I had no ready reply to their accusations of vanity.

When I was almost ten, my family moved from a mostly white section of D.C. to a similarly homogenous section of a northern New Jersey suburb, where I stayed until I left for college. I must have been about thirteen when I became friends with two sisters, one my age and one a couple of years older. They introduced me to the comforting sounds of The Smiths, The Cure, and other postpunk British artists who seemed as internally embattled as I was. I found the music cheerful; there was a club of beautiful outcasts that I could potentially join if I learned the rules. The sisters shopped at Goodwill but wore expensive Doc Marten boots, lots of makeup, and silver jewelry. Soon I had outfitted myself in comparable garb and assimilated the aesthetic: Siouxsie Sioux, vampire pale. I wouldn't leave my house without a layer of whitish powder smoothed across my face and blood-red lipstick coating my lips. I plucked my eyebrows into thin arcs, bleached my mustache, and tried to look as corpselike as possible. Sometimes, at home by myself, I'd think I looked okay. But the next time I'd check the girls' bathroom mirror at school, nothing would be where I'd left it. My eyebrows would seem overplucked, my forehead would have shrunken under my low, encroaching hairline, and my nose would loom before me like the ultimate betrayal. After school, I'd spend hours staring at pictures of my favorite porcelain pop stars or hanging out with my new goth friends, eating the junk food I was forbidden to eat at home and watching old episodes of MTV's *120 Minutes.*

For all those hours, days, and years, I indulged myself as best I could in a fantasy of whiteness. I tried not to think about what I looked like, tried not to look, but then couldn't resist. Over time, the shock dulled, and I became resigned to my fate.

I know now that I was not the only brownish person who felt ugly growing up in a white milieu. As an adult living in Queens, New York, I've made many friends who happen to have one white parent and one parent whose skin is some shade of brown. They have stories that I recognize as versions of my own school years, stories of wishing they were white. We laughed when we confessed that each of us had one body part in particular that we felt placed us beyond any hope of blending in, that we'd have done almost anything to alter. And we timidly told stories of how we stayed away from the few other minority kids—who existed at the margins of an elementary school—because the last thing we wanted was to be confused for one of them, especially the immigrants. For those of us born here, who could speak the language and reference the culture with the ease of our white American counterparts, emulating the white kids was a compelling yet elusive game. We were almost like our peers, but never quite. Never able to actually be white.

My game of chasing whiteness came to an abrupt end on September 11, 2001. The air was charged with potential, for peace and for war. But for Arabs and Muslims, or anyone who *looked* Arab or Muslim, the possibilities were closing in fast: suspect, target, victim. I was lucky; the harassment I faced left no visible mark on my body, and because I was born in America, I couldn't easily be detained or deported like thousands of others. But I listened as my coworkers demanded revenge.

"We should bomb Iraq and Iran, bomb the whole place," one of them said, and no one disagreed.

Hearing this that tragic morning, too stunned to speak, I remembered that I had family in Iran whom I'd never met, whose names I didn't even know. A few days later, I was on my way to an anti-war organizing meeting when I was stopped by a New York City police officer, for what reason she wouldn't say, but we both knew it had to do with my suspicious-looking face.

At anti-war events, I was asked to speak as a woman of color, as an Iranian American, for the first time. There was no confusion about how other people saw me; the question now was how I would see myself. When I watched a tall, red-faced man yell at a Muslim woman on 23rd Street—indignant that she would flaunt her religion by covering her head at a time like this—I identified so fully with her that I felt as if what was happening to her was also happening to me, that we had both been threatened with an unpredictable rage that had come unhinged. After all, those who commit hate crimes rarely stop to check if you are actually what they think you are.

No longer able to avoid my Iranian heritage, I had to make it into something more than a reason to feel vulnerable and powerless, something more than simply another kind of erasure. And I began to realize how much I'd already lost, how many years of learning about Iranian culture and history, of speaking Persian, of visiting Iran, of being a part of my family there. But most of all, I missed my father, missed all the years when we might have been close, might have been proud to be Iranian together. I felt empty and full of longing at the same time. When I looked in the bathroom mirror of my Queens apartment, I realized I was incapable of accurately interpreting the image before me. The most insidious part of assimilation is the way it has distorted my vision, mangled my face, and made me push my brown relatives away.

More than two years later, in the winter of 2004, I made my first trip to Iran, alone, and on a one-way ticket. After all the bureaucratic hurdles and the months it took to get in touch with my father's family in Teheran, after a lifetime apart, I wanted to stay as long as I could. From the moment of my arrival at the gates of Mehrabad Airport, I began assimilating a new landscape of faces. One by one, members of my extended family came into focus, as if they were each stepping out from behind a curtain of anonymity on cue. My cousin Raha, my uncle's daughter, saw me first, and in an instant, I was picked out of the crowd and claimed. She was a taller, more broadly framed woman than I (lovingly nicknamed Bulldozer by her husband, as I would later learn, because she had survived a series of grave illnesses and proven to be indestructible), but I could find my face in hers. Something radiating from her tea-colored eyes and smiling pink lips bound us together, held me steady. She reached for me and tried to kiss each of my cheeks while I tried to hug her. I was already getting the ritual of greeting wrong, but there was no time to dwell or to doubt. My uncle was there, waiting to greet me.

My father's only brother looked like a shorter, older version of my father, with deep brown skin, a slight build, and thin white hair that was receding, unlike my father's, which was still thick and bushy and out of control. He was clean shaven, also like my father, and his simple light blue shirt, navy blue sweater, and gray suit looked old and worn. I wanted to tell him that he and my father dress alike, even though they've lived apart for close to fifty years, that it seemed as if it were some brotherly uniform. But my fledgling Persian kept me from any outbursts of recognition, limiting my speech to a series of *Salaams*.

My uncle's wife said things to me I didn't understand. She had a wrinkled old-woman's face with pale skin and a pointy nose. I couldn't see her properly that first day because of the scarf and shawl draped over her head, hanging down the front of her long black winter coat. I couldn't see the 1960s-style flip in her hair or her shapely legs. It's a funny way to meet people for the first time, all covered up. Well, only the women, of course. It would take me weeks to see the traces of how beautiful she must have been once, and months before she would be beautiful to me.

Raha's husband, Hami, was a slightly plump man of medium height. He leaned on a crutch, his left foot in a cast. His dark, wavy hair matched his mustache and gave his round face a boyish look. Exhaustion conspired to age him prematurely, slackening his features and turning the whites of his eyes red. He smiled with some effort, like he was rising to the occasion.

A darting movement drew my gaze downward. Golnar, Raha and Hami's older daughter, poked her head out from behind her mother's coat with the hesitant anticipation of a seven-year-old. *Can I come out? Can I show you who I am?* Her short, playful brown curls showed off her round face and enormous brown eyes. She was a chubby kid with that irresistible quality that marked her for much cheek pinching. Only then did I see the bundle in my uncle's wife's arms, at first indistinguishable to me from her layers of hand-knitted shawls: Hediyeh, Golnar's five-month-old sister. She looked like her father: a miniature, baby-girl version of Hami's round face, bundled up against the winter chill. Hediyeh's first winter in Teheran. She and I would share many firsts that year.

Over the next six months, I would negotiate my place among this multigenerational family, living together under one roof. And I would learn my way around the city, make it my own by choosing favorites from among the many cafés and tea-houses, by deciding upon the most idyllic picnic spot, the tastiest cheap–lunch joint, the quietest and quaintest alleyways, and by returning to them all again and again.

When I walked down the tree-lined streets of Teheran, with the creeklike trickle of rainwater keeping pace alongside me below the curb like a constant companion, I wore a thin black manteau that stopped at mid-thigh, and a gold and magenta silk scarf wrapped around my head. My scarf looked more like a bonnet, tied tightly in place beneath my chin, compared with the scarves of the women who had grown up in Iran and managed elegant draping effects reminiscent of 1950s movie stars. What we had in common was that every inch of every curve of our bodies was not on display. As I moved through my days, up and down Vali-Asr Boulevard between my Persian language classes and my uncle's house, those flattened, beckoning women I had become accustomed to seeing in New York were not leaning seductively down at me from billboards or calling out to me from magazine kiosks. I began to walk away from the constant battle for perfection that trains us to chop up our faces and bodies into "good" and "bad" parts. I stopped carrying a mirror in my bag.

I was a stranger surrounded by strangers, but the feeling of blending into the crowds on Teheran's broad avenues was like luxuriating in the familiar, novel though it was. My skin, my hair, my face were reflected back to me in infinite variation, until I was just another Iranian woman walking down the street, unremarkable as long as I kept quiet and didn't reveal my American accent. And my face, my presence, seemed to brighten up my uncle's household, to break up the routine. My cousins and I grew so fond of each other that we often rushed through our separate daily activities, distracted and anxious, until we were reunited in the evenings.

Fridays, when schools and businesses closed, were like private celebrations. My uncle's wife would cook one of my favorite meat-and-rice dishes with a savory fruit or with pomegranate paste, unless it was one of the special days each month when Zoroastrians are forbidden to eat meat. On those days, set aside to prevent humans from depleting nature's bounty, we ate eggplant frittatas or lentil stews. Raha and my other cousin Khodadad would take turns singing old Persian love songs they'd grown up listening to on their parents' turntable. The first time one of them asked me to "sing a poem," I was speechless until I realized the words for "sing" and "read," "poem" and "song," are interchangeable. They'd never heard of The Smiths or The Cure, but my cousins loved Madonna and clamored for a rendition of "Like a Prayer." Having never seen the video, and unable to decipher most of the lyrics beyond the title, they thought it was a purely pious song, uncomplicated by carnal passions. I obliged as best I could, unable to explain the other, earthly subtext even if I'd wanted to. I didn't know those kinds of words. At some point during the festivities, my uncle would turn the floor over to Golnar, who would perform the little songs and dances she'd memorized in kindergarten.

I'd been part of these gatherings for less than three months when it happened—when I recognized my face as something benign, something good. I was stuffed into the living room along with my father's brother and sister, six of my cousins and their many children—a room made even more crowded by the voices of three generations talking over and to each other, cracking jokes and telling stories that would become incomprehensible to me as soon as the speaker got carried away, picking up speed and busting up sentences with irrepressible laughter. Teacups in saucers balanced on every available surface, and delicate china plates sat in irregular piles with half-eaten pastries, fruit-peel shavings, and small mountains of sunflower-seed shells wedged in between them. A cousin asked me to weigh in on what had become a debate about why Iran's future looked so bleak. I was in the middle of a sentence when I arrived at that inevitable stopping point again, unable to say what I felt I must say in my fledgling Persian. Thirty-year-old carpets cushioned my feet as I rose to go find my dictionary. There, in the cramped back bedroom stuffed with the accumulated possessions of my extended family, artifacts of the years up until now, before our paths crossed, I found something beautiful in that graying, square mirror affixed to the back of the door.

Snagged by my own reflection, I stopped and stared. Nothing jarred. Nothing tweaked my consciousness painfully away from some imagined, whiter version of myself. It was as if the settings in my brain had changed and reconfigured what my mind could see. And I thought, *Oh, so that's what I look like.* I heard myself sigh in relief. Nothing was ugly or needed to be changed. There was nothing American, Jewish, Zoroastrian, or Iranian to hate or to hide. I laughed with myself. I smiled, and it was me I saw smiling. Then I knew what it meant to feel at home.

And yet, I still felt out of sync. It seemed like I was the only woman in the Islamic Republic who was experiencing some kind of individual liberation. While I reveled in the respite from my self-consciousness, in the absence of white Westerners and the graphic American-style sexism I was used to ingesting—letting my eyebrows grow out and deciding I no longer needed to be quite so skinny—something very different seemed to be underway for the resident population. Iran for Iranian women didn't seem to offer the same possibility for an embrace of one's unaltered, actual self that I was able to contemplate. I took to counting the number of times a day I saw a man or woman walking down the busy streets with a bandage over his or her nose. This indicated he or she was recovering from a recent nose job, a status symbol among the Teherani hipsters. One day I counted twelve. There was speculation that some bandages were fakes, ploys to convince others that the wearer was wealthy enough to have indulged in this trendy import from the West. I understood the logic that drove this defacing craze; I grew up wanting a nose job too. I used to stare at myself in my bedroom mirror, pushing my nose up ever so slightly with my pointer finger, and think, *There. Just like that. That would be perfect.*

Iranian women have their eyebrows threaded at younger ages than ever before, and their makeup is getting thicker and more obvious, much to the chagrin of the older generation, who generally think it appropriate to beautify oneself only after a marriage engagement has been secured. The headscarves reveal more and more bleached blond and highlighted hair; the manteaus have grown tighter, shorter, and more transparent. This is part of a social rebellion; the form-fitting clothes and lavish cosmetics undermine regime dictates—something that obviously can't be said about comparably provocative attire in the United States.

But what kind of liberation will this bring? When I looked into the glamorous faces of the Iranian women I passed on the streets, I felt the urge to judge myself shabby and unkempt by comparison. But I didn't. I thought I saw a layer of strain underneath all that makeup. These women were simultaneously held to two rigid sets of rules—one official, and one imported. There's a global conception of feminine beauty, standardized by the West even here. It's the same "striving toward Barbie" ideal I know too well, oddly positioned in Iran as an act of resistance against the shapeless black chadors of religious Shi'ism. But covered or uncovered, it seems to me, the complex subjectivity of women can still remain invisible. If the choices are between the rule of the clerics and the rule of the beauty industries, how will we ever gain real control over our lives, or over how we see ourselves?

After six months at my uncle's house, it was time to go home, back to Queens, to my friends and my life as a political activist. But I was also going back to try something new with the fractured nuclear family I'd left behind. I'd learned something from my uncle, his wife, their children and grandchildren—something about how to love my own people and how to stop battling against myself. My hope was that this experience would translate into my relationships with my father, my mother, and my sister; that I could see them as differently as I now saw myself.

I lay awake on my last night, contemplating my return. *You mustn't lose yourself again,* I warned. The metal frame of my small bed registered my worry with its squeaky refrain. I tossed and turned, wrestling with the wary knowledge that I might not be able to withstand the visual onslaught awaiting me back home. Would I succumb to the old confusion, to that distorted vision that hid me from myself like no hijab ever could? I squeezed my eyes tighter, trying to stop the unsettling thoughts. Inside the blackness, there was something solid and calm I could grab on to, the sensation that infused my soul when I found myself in that mirror. *I'm still me. I'm always me. Hold on to this. Remember.* I wished the coherence, the face, I'd found was like a souvenir that I could clutch in my pocket the whole way home; that I could gaze at unaltered anytime I chose. But I knew it wasn't. I was falling through darkness away from myself, already missing my Iranian family, asleep in the adjacent rooms, and who I had been among them.

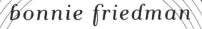

bonnie friedman

BEAUTY
FROM THE
UNDERWORLD

*At the age of forty-one, I
became visible. I was drawn,
briefly, to a man who cared how I
looked.* Up until then, being inconspicuous—even libera-
tingly unkempt—was native to me. I shuffled around the
neighborhood in smudged glasses and my husband's big green
puffy pants, half submerged in the scenes I'd been writing,
blinking at my neighbors through smeared fingerprints. Only
on the rarest of occasions did I wear makeup. Mostly the stuff
lay stowed in the linen closet, where it turned as cracked and
hard as watercolor tiles in its blue-floral tea cozy of a bag—a
pouch with a sprung wire that scratched my hands whenever
I reached for a pillowcase. Even on Saturday night, when
my husband and I went out, I usually wore the trousers his
mother gave me for Hanukkah—high-waisted, perma-press
affairs with an almost comical button floating above my

navel and falling in billowing columns over my toes. My hair was a dark, chopped edge.

The truth was that my husband and I were benignly oblivious to how I looked. What counted was who I was—what I thought and said. We'd met in college. I'd revered feminists and intellectuals—Susan Sontag with her skunk streak and bulky sweaters, Gloria Steinem with her unstained face as honest as raw pine. Concern for one's appearance reflected, I believed, a sort of spiritual malady as debilitating as a limp.

But then came this flirtation, this captivation and rearrangement of my internal electrical field, and suddenly I owned a silvery Lycra skirt and leather boots, and I stood hyperventilating in Sephora on Prince Street, inhaling the whirl of perfumes whose backlit bottles resided on pedestals along the darkened walls like icons of Eros, like the golden nectar of glamour itself—oh, if only I could sip it! If only I could draw that elixir of beauty permanently into me! For, having become aware that in certain contexts I might actually appear beautiful, having discovered that beauty wasn't only for the moronically superficial or congenitally lucky (as I'd heretofore convinced myself), and having discovered, furthermore, what it felt like to be seen, to have craved eyes upon me, I had, at the same time and to my vast dismay, discovered my own abundant physical flaws: the wrinkles etched in my forehead, the age spot set like an asterisk above my right eye.

Now I wandered up and down the twinkling aisles, unsure of what to buy and wishing that I could seize it all, that I could retrieve the magical box of beauty as Psyche had been commanded to do when she traveled to the underworld. Ultimately,

I bought four or five things; the prices alone were dazzling. My bounty included a translucent face powder, like faintly lustrous skin pollen, and a mocha Vincent Longo lipstick that seemed an emblem of sultry, confident femininity. Then home I went.

Could I look, here, as I had in the glittering emporium? Or did the urbane face live only there? As it turned out, it did not—amazingly. I had brought that face home with me. The stuff worked. My appearance transformed. I saw myself as that man seemed to. But why had I believed that I was lackluster for so long? It was as if I'd lived under the spell of an old hypnosis. I was not longer the girl I'd been for forty-one years (somehow, I'd remained a girl all that time). The mirror showed a woman with a plush mouth, cheekbones, and blue eyes that knew a secret I didn't. I tossed out the old stuff—teal shadow, candy-pink rouge, Cyndi Lauper colors I'd bought at Sears fifteen years earlier and that now seemed like the touch-up hues on a rotogravure. I threw out the tea-cozy bag too, with its crabbed, stabbing wire like a defective brassiere, for it seemed like the repository of an old concept of myself, one in which I was a plain, dutiful, invisible girl, someone sisterly or maternal, engulfed by a kind of furniture cover of sturdy, dull fabric that I'd assumed constituted myself.

For the next three weeks, I was a girl in a pointillist painting—shimmering, thrilled, my skin a skein of electric dots and dashes trying to signal to me something to which, for half my life, I'd been oblivious. I bought an eyelash clamp. I pierced my ears. On the subway I stared at the exquisite plum-glossed lips of an Asian girl. Where had she found that tint? Another woman had fascinating eyebrows—thick, plush. *The brows are the frames of the face,* I repeated to myself, a dictum just discovered in a makeup book.

I wanted, I wanted—to be looked at, to be seen. Oh, to be beautiful! I'd always assumed that the superficial was of only superficial importance, not that one's soul glimmered across one's skin. Now, at forty-one, it seemed otherwise. I became one of the appearance-obsessed, studying *Hair Style* magazine at Barnes & Noble. How did Jennifer Aniston do that thing? I must have been the last woman in America to ask.

Everywhere I looked, beauty glimmered as if it had been rained over the city and was vanishing down a thousand grates. Exquisite women slipped out the subway doors, strode off elevators, stepped into the wheeling glass compartments of revolving doors, as if beauty itself were always disappearing—a seduction, a promise, a yearning, a lack. I was left contemplating an odd collection of features I coveted: lips, brows, eyelids, feet. All I wanted to do was shop. I couldn't sit still at my desk long enough to think. And my writing had hardened, clumping into garlands of verbiage. I could no longer vanish down the rabbit hole of words. How foolish my work seemed! Make-believe, intellectualization. What mattered was the body.

"You look great," said the man who cared about my appearance. He stared, smiling, and drew the cigarette from his lips.

But unease flared inside me. My guilt at indulging this flirtation grew ever more acute. And I could not really believe that my years of invisibility had been wasted. After all, they'd been full of intellectual adventures that had brought truths. I missed being able to think. My marriage, too, was marvelous in so many ways. I loved and adored my husband, and felt known by him. Yet what should I make of the shocking discovery that you can be drawn to the surface of yourself, like fish rushing to the surface when food is sprinkled? I seemed to contain a thousand mouths.

My personality felt kidnapped. I was at war with myself. *Appearance does not matter*, my heels banged out, even as I dashed back to the mirror to see which face peered back at me. Would it be the familiar round homey old one? Or the long new one with the knowing eyes, the one I found "beautiful"? But the mirror figure floating in a matching but backward bathroom wouldn't say. After a month, I cut off contact with the man who told me he liked my looks. But I was left no longer really even knowing my own hair color. Was it chestnut, veined with gray? Or was it the blond I'd found at the salon? Was I somehow still beautiful, as I'd momentarily been? I recalled the first patient of talk therapy, Sophie F., described in *Studies in Hysteria*. She'd looked down at her brown dress and called it blue, her eyes seeing the dress she'd worn exactly a week earlier. In fact, she often perceived herself as wearing what she had exactly seven days before, her brain exposing old images, her eyes seeing herself clad in the past.

I couldn't sort myself either. Sometimes my husband said, with an indulgent smile, "You're wearing makeup!" It made me feel like some dear, pathetic creature who'd made an effort. I lived again in my big green pants. But I wondered constantly about that giddy woman who stood across Lexington Avenue in a short black dress, pulse banging in her wrists and up her arms, feeling gorgeous. I'd never met her before and yet she sprang out of me, and now she was gone and I missed her, although her dress hung in my closet.

Could I get her beauty back? How? The answer was not in the mirror or at Sephora or in the underworld of transgression, which, in New York, runs as continually as the subways. Beauty lived in the eye of the beholder, and my beholder was gone. In my ears rang a childhood rhyme: "Lucy Locket has lost her pocket and doesn't know where to find it." I felt like Lucy Locket.

I met my husband during my senior year of college. On weekends we cooked omelets, which seemed exotic then, throwing in green peppers, onions, Monterey Jack cheese, cracked black pepper, and mushrooms, and then clamping a lid on top while the whole thing rose in its cast-iron skillet over a steady flame, quadrupling in size into a frothy, delectable wheel so big it seemed some beneficent force must be adding ingredients under the tight lid. We sat at a picnic table in his back yard and ate for hours, talking about everything, getting up to saw off slices of the yeast bread his housemate baked and smearing them with the butter that lived on the kitchen table on a plate. He was a grand storyteller, full of tales of Berkeley, where he'd lived during a semester off, surviving on the popcorn at the movie theater where he changed the marquee, singing in Spanish at the Cheesecake Factory, where all his coworkers were Mexican, making his own way. When he told stories, leaning toward me across the table, describing subtleties of texture and tone, I felt lucky. What gifts of perception and expression he possessed! It felt like the gateway to a marvelous intimacy.

After we married, I wondered if Augustine was right and it was blasphemy to love my husband so much. A Georgia O'Keeffe painting, borrowed from the library, hung on the wall opposite our bed. It had big white-iron petals and a pollen-plush center. Checking out art from the library had been my husband's idea. I liked knowing that each canvas had a brown envelope glued invisibly to its back. It seemed like a secret connection to a private world, a little pouch of self tucked from view, happy evidence that we'd made use of the resources at hand. And it seemed typical of my husband to discover and be game for this fun thing—art borrowing! The view from our bed changed every two months, and I even liked toting the framed print back to the library, because then we could chose something else— purple and blue Chagalls with floating brides, Paul Klee fish, Miró moons and hooks and eyelike emblems—a catalog of dreams, a secret language we loved but didn't understand, and which beckoned like our own future.

In Brooklyn, years later, my husband was still extravagantly wonderful company, but something seemed lacking. Often I felt I could be anyone tagging along beside him. I felt like a sidekick, a pal, a good affectionate dog standing on my hind legs to lick his face. At a friend's wedding, my husband and I found ourselves sitting on the lush green lawn with a woman whose own husband had stayed home. While my husband spoke, this woman smiled. Her head bobbed eagerly as if on a spring, and her smile of delight seemed both sincere and yet set in place. My husband grew expansive; he seemed excited, brimming with joy. *I could be her*, I thought. *She could replace me, and I could just step away. What my husband needs is a smiling, receptive woman—it never needed to be me.* This thought was both devastating and liberating.

Not long after, I met the man who liked how I looked. And now that he was gone, I no longer could return to my old inconspicuousness, for it felt no longer like invisibility, but like ugliness.

"I need you to let me know. Do you like how I look?" I asked my husband.

"Yup," he said. "You look good all the time."

"Well, if you think it, tell me."

But he almost never did. He'd come from a family where compliments were rare, and sarcasm frequent.

And now, without the mirror of that other man's eyes, my own sense of self started to depart like the pupil of a person going wall-eyed. One part of me felt twisted away, while another stared straight ahead. Things had too many dimensions or too few. I craved to once again be that beautiful girl I'd been, but didn't want to leave my marriage. It seemed my beauty lived on the staircase to that man's office; the higher I ascended it, the more beautiful I became, until his eyes saw me and the transformation was complete. But this was filching beauty, shoplifting love, behaving like someone feral, desperate, undeserving, nasty within. I couldn't do it anymore. Nor could I pick up my home life where I'd left off.

In her trip from the underworld with her box of beauty, Psyche breaks the rules. She was supposed to hand the package from the goddess of Hades straight into the hands of Venus—no looking inside! But, overcome with curiosity, she opens the lid and falls into a deathlike sleep. Because the box doesn't contain beauty. No. It contains a cargo of jinxed slumber, a poppy field in a box, and Psyche collapses dead in her tracks until Eros awakens her. I'd been asleep too, under my pot lid, cozy, shut away in my cubicle, beguiling myself with complicated thoughts, not suspecting I was becoming like the professor in *Strange Interlude*—"a refugee from reality." The snug, safe, pot-lid life suited me. The fire of my stove was warm, and it was nice to have armor all around. But that life no longer worked. You can't happily choose an existence that you now realize is an opiated stasis. I could not happily shut my cubicle door. The world kept calling my name—in the way a woman and a man kissed on the 5 train, in the smile a husband gave his wife in front of a brownstone down the street. Longing stretched within me, then snapped with a horrible pang.

I began attending Codependents Anonymous, a twelve-step group that met in a hospital. I wasn't quite sure why I'd come. An acquaintance with sympathetic eyes had gone away for two weeks to Italy. We'd sent each other some emails and had lunch once. But I felt devastated, abandoned, as if life now had no meaning. Obviously this was a wild, mad, berserk overreaction to his departure, as I informed myself while I wept. It was August in New York; only a few solitary figures moved down the blistering streets. A hot white sun pulsed in a gluey sky. Life was elsewhere. I thought of the dental phenomenon of "referred pain," where one tooth is decayed but a different tooth hurts. I recalled the endodontist coming at me with a big gray ice cube held with tongs. "It's the only way we can really determine where the pain is coming from," he said as he pushed the ice cube into my mouth. "Here?" he said, sliding the ice. "Here?" I rocketed out of the seat, pain blazing to the root of my heels, then throbbing with a long half-life.

"See? It wasn't the tooth you came in pointing to," he explained kindly to my leaky eyes.

I supposed this Italy-bound man had inadvertently touched some integral, irrational hurt. And I wanted to feel more in control of my life. I wanted to feel less needy. I didn't like the idea of a man I barely knew going away and making me feel he'd pulled all the meaning of life after him, like a person turning in bed, obliviously taking the blankets. So I started attending these meetings, which had everything to do with getting free from psychological enslavement. Beneath the hospital's fluorescent lights, our skin glinted like sandpaper, and we all seemed to be wearing dingy thrift-shop jeans and sneakers that had lost their tread—a gathering of the marginal, the peripheral, the figures who lurk in the corner of one's eye. More than our actual clothing, though, the way we looked seemed an effect of the bleaching, granular tube lights of the hospital.

In the beginning I told myself, *This isn't really me*, as I've often told myself at beginnings. We went around the circle, and each person spoke for four minutes. It was all anonymous except for your first name. Stories of remote or impervious partners, of perfectionist parents and parents who'd vanished into addictions, of choosing as lovers people interred in sadness or anger or marriage to someone else, of compulsively trying to control one's environment (I thought of my pot lid) or other people (I thought of the truths I'd never shared with my husband for fear of his reaction, and because if I said them, they'd seem real). And there were other stories too, of marvelous dancing, of reading to a daughter *The Little Engine That Could*, of spontaneous poetry and hard-earned restraint. Aria after aria, each four minutes long, and I sang my aria too. Odd that this maskless, cruelly lit place is where I began to rediscover my sense of beauty.

"Hi, Bonnie," said a few of the people in the group when I came to my third or fourth meeting. I blinked, surprised they knew my name. I seemed to believe I was always shucking off the husk of myself, as if my real self were metamorphosing faster than any of us could register, and it was always only the old clothing of myself—already disavowed—that others could see. This was a defense, of course. The people here connected me to what I'd said before; they were accumulating me, the truest parts of me, and didn't forget me from week to week.

After the meeting, I walked west on light rubber heels, past two hushed green parks and a chapel where a gospel chorus sang to empty pews, the windows thrown open. Often I stopped to listen. The city no longer felt populated by strangers, because I was hearing so many other people's secrets. Everyone was a hidden envelope, a tucked-away pouch. On the subway I was calmer, and if my eyes met those of a weary woman across the aisle, or of a father soothing his child, we exchanged a smile. People no longer seemed so alien and scary and insubstantial, and neither did I.

And then I started wearing the clothing I'd bought during my carnival time. A short suede skirt. A tight green top. The faux-alligator boots. My husband smiled, a private appraising smile. "All dressed up," he might say. "Mmm-hmm," I'd respond. I often wore a silver bracelet I'd bought in Arizona. This bracelet felt like a totem, something lucky and magical. It reminded me of something about myself. I no longer implored my husband to make me feel beautiful. Sometimes he did, and then it was as if we shared a secret between us, a private energy field, with the current glinting back and forth. Sometimes he didn't, and then I could tell the secret to myself, glancing at the bracelet and remembering a blanket spread on the red earth in Arizona, the Native American woman with silver baubles that could be trinkets or treasures. Their value was what you saw in them. I'd bought this bracelet for $10, and when my glance fell on it, a blessing seemed to flash up, a wink.

Now I no longer felt invisible. A mirror had somehow gotten propped up inside. I existed, occasionally smart, often stupid, but more and more real. I could see now that my husband was basically shy about compliments; it didn't mean he didn't see me. Having longed to be seen by his own parents, who'd ignored him almost on principle, he wasn't at ease giving praise. I learned to notice his more subtle signals—his glinting, sunny gaze, the nod of approval when I stood up for myself, the way he brought me a sack of apricot-centered butter cookies he'd bought because he knew I adored them, the way he gave me the window seat on railroad trips so I had the better view.

These days it seems to me that the body is a purse clasping the soul of the self, and the soul is always changing. Its nature is metamorphosis. It can't stay in its cubicle cocoon forever without withering. We betray ourselves if we don't set forth. Now, teaching a class, riding the subway, my glance falls on my bracelet, and a reassuring gleam winks up from it—a last echo of the man who cared how I looked, and a reminder of my husband's real love for my particular company, and of the girl whose desire for beauty was long locked away, a secret even from herself.

kamy wicoff

COMING OUT OF THE CURLY CLOSET:

CONFESSIONS OF A BLOWOUT QUEEN

I don't spend a lot of time in front of a mirror looking at my face. Actually, that's not true. I spend a lot of time in front of a mirror looking at my face. But I am always *doing* something to it—covering up the purplish bags under my eyes with concealer, jutting my chin toward the mirror and narrowing my eyes like a gangster as I apply mascara, or, if I'm feeling really ambitious, attempting to dab liquidy black eyeliner onto the inner rim of my upper eyelids. I learned this method from a Make-up Artist, who made sure to tell me that she was, in fact, an artist, and who drew such convincing analogies between painting art and painting your face that she managed to sell me enough never-since-used make-up brushes to make myself into the Incredible Hulk. Other activities include baring my gums to floss or examining a new freckle. I certainly never get close enough to the mirror to see things I don't feel like seeing, and I steer clear of the mirrors that magnify every pore, like the one my Aunt Patsy gave me when I was eleven, designed by Conair, with light settings DAY, OFFICE, EVENING, and HOME.

I haven't always been this way. The Christmas day that Aunt Patsy gave me the Conair mirror, I set it up immediately, pulling each of its hinged side mirrors toward my cheeks to form a tiny chapel, sat down on my vanity chair with the shiny metal heart-shaped back and white vinyl cushioned seat (it was a tacky chair, but in my fantasies it transported me to the land of one hundred brushstrokes, the courtesan's boudoir), tucked my legs under the mustard-colored Formica bathroom counter, and proceeded to sit and stare at my face. For hours. I had the enormous luxury, or misfortune, to have acquired my own bathroom when my family moved into a bigger subdivision and a bigger house. Sitting and staring at my face became a ritual, usually after school, sometimes before bed. For the most part, I was trying to figure out what was wrong with it. There were a lot of possibilities. I had a big nose. I had braces. I had moles. I particularly hated the moles. "Mole" was one of those words—like "mustache," "armpit hair," or "bad breath"—that an eleven year old girl never wanted to hear uttered in reference to her appearance, but that my sixth-grade "friends" used very frequently when picking apart my unsatisfactory appearance loudly and pointedly every day at lunch.

Staring at my face in those days, however—even under the harsh light of OFFICE—did me little good. My blue eyes were clearly my best feature, but I could not walk around all day with my nose and chin tucked into my elbow, like Dracula, though

I often tried this while sitting at my desk. I knew of no beauty treatments in San Antonio more radical than hair highlights and tanning beds—both out of my price range and my parents' willingness to support. In my desperation to be tan (which, ironically, multiplied the moles considerably), I used to drag a perennially dirt-encrusted tan-and-orange lawn chair, a few of its vinyl slats unattached in inopportune places, to the only sunny strip of our tree-crammed back yard. This also happened to be the home of the giant, industrial-green, deafening air-conditioning compressor, tasked with blowing all the hot air out of the house. It was hell, even with my extension cord, boom box, iced tea, and fan. But I did it, sweating and flipping, because a tan was something I could actually acquire on my own.

Tan or pale, however, I knew I was stuck with my face—though later, when I was fourteen or fifteen, Aunt Patsy did offer to pay for a nose job. (I declined, finally beginning to believe my mother's passionate arguments that my big nose gave my face "character.") But even before this intriguing and insulting offer, the knowledge that I was stuck with my face forced me to make peace with it. The truth was, it really wasn't that bad, especially when I turned the knob to EVENING and gave myself a break. In those moods, my hours in front of that Conair mirror flickered with hope. In my face I could see possibility, could drift away into a foreseeable future, where beauty came to me with maturity and time—contingent, of course, on a key move to a state where former Dallas Cowboys cheerleaders and Linda Evans wannabes were not the paragons of hotness at PTA meetings and the neighborhood pool. But it wasn't long until I found a way to disrupt this fantasy completely. With determination and desperation, fueled by my continuing lack of success as an attractive girl at school, another key part of my appearance supplanted my face as my mortal enemy: my hair. At twelve, my hair became the first thing I looked at in the mirror—and the first thing I loathed with the hysterical passion of which twelve-year-old girls are uniquely capable.

In my mind, there was only one major problem with my hair, but it was huge: It was curly, and I hated it. Perhaps because I was a blond-haired, blue-eyed girl with curly hair, I hated it even more. Like every girl in Texas, I had absorbed the Barbie beauty ideal (ripping the long, straight, shiny hair out of Barbies' rubber scalps was minimally therapeutic), and with an unconscious bigotry I am ashamed to admit to, I probably felt I was *entitled* to have the locks of a WASPy white girl and had been unfairly deprived of them. Soon, when I looked into my Conair mirror, I pulled my hair away from my face so tightly that my eyes smarted with tears, and I took masochistic pleasure in the pain this caused me. It was satisfying both to punish my hair and to vent the visceral outrage I felt at its very existence on my head.

This may seem extreme, but growing up female in Texas in the 1980s *was* extreme. Especially in the hair department. Hair was king. (Think *Dallas*.) Hair was big. Hair was straight (elementary school), and then it was permed (junior high). My hair was curly, which meant it had never been straight and would never look permed, because curly hair and permed hair, as everyone knows, are two totally different things. The pouting, woeful sigh Molly Ringwald directed at her small tits in *Sixteen Candles* was a quaint and tame depiction compared with the kind of fury I directed at my mane. I did not sigh about my hair; I yelled at it. In moments of steely control, I talked calmly to it, as you would to a crazy person. I pulled at it until I cried—yanked at it, cursed it, and occasionally actually tore it out; wet it, Aqua Netted it, gelled it, braided it, curling-ironed it, cut it, singed it (along with my forehead)—and nothing made it look right.

Looking back at this period now, from the wise old vantage point of thirty-five, I can laugh. Sort of. At least I can see the bigger picture. My hair was bad, yes. At its worst—when gigantic, valley-girl bangs were the hairstyle everyone had to have—my unruly curls caused my attempt at big bangs to collapse in the clutches of Texas humidity as soon as I walked out my door, stickily sagging downward like an ill-placed toupee about to lose its grip on my forehead. This would frustrate anyone. To stomp my feet, talk to myself, scream, and mutilate the hair on my own head, however—leading my mother to maintain a cautious but steadfast distance from the door of my bathroom each morning—was crazy. But it was not abnormal. As Mary Pipher observed in *Reviving Ophelia*, the average twelve-year-old girl should be thought about like a person perpetually on acid. Not because the average twelve-year-old girl is crazy, but because she is reacting to a crazy system. In my case, this system made me feel that a girl's place in the social hierarchy of the world was determined almost solely by the way she looked, and my ineptitude in this department (and my bad hair!) was to blame for casting me down to the bottom and placing a bunch of stupid, petty, eerily serene, and frequently mean girls at the top. I wanted to be beautiful, because as far as I could see, being beautiful meant being powerful; it meant not getting kicked around, as unpretty girls are.

My fantasies of becoming beautiful someday were shaped accordingly: In the romantic comedy/makeover movie starring me, I never responded to the miracle of transforming into a knockout with demure humility or adorable, hesitant confusion—as heroines as ancient as Cinderella or as close to me as Ally Sheedy in *The Breakfast Club* had always done. The makeover movie I mentally starred in when I was in junior high was much closer to a comic-book adaptation than to a chick flick. In it, I played the role of the demented villain, who in the climactic scene stood under the superpowered gorgeousness gamma ray I'd invented after years of laboring alone in my ugly cave, flipped the switch, and threw my head back in triumph as I greedily soaked up every bit of that female steroid: hotness. I then wreaked havoc with my new powers on every boy, girl, and grownup who had ever slandered me, pitied me, ignored me, or danced around me in a circle, chanting, "Witch nose, curly hair."

Now is the part where I am supposed to say that I have completely outgrown this fantasy. That when I retired my Conair mirror, I made peace with my curly hair too, and that I now look in the mirror and gaze at my natural curls with mature benignity. I would love to say that—especially now that I am a mother of two little boys, and hypothetically I should know that there are much more important things for me to spend my time doing than battling with my hair. But I can't. Because when I was twenty-two (why did she wait so long!?), good old Aunt Patsy clued me in to a hairstyling regimen I'd had no idea existed, but now cannot leave my house without: the blowout. With a hairdryer, a round bristle brush, strong forearm muscles, and some time, I can go from being a curly-headed woman out of the shower to being a straight-haired woman on the street. Talk about a miracle!

I don't spend a lot of time in front of a mirror, looking at my face. But every day I spend about fifteen minutes, or twenty, or sometimes (gulp!) twenty-five, depending on how humid it is, standing in front of a mirror, staring at my hair. And at least once, every single time I do it, the question enters my head: *Am I still stuck in the seventh grade?* With a few exceptions, however, this question has yet to stop me.

My first blowout was like standing under the beauty gamma ray. It wasn't easy to endure. My head was yanked firmly from side to side by a stylist wielding a tough, round, boar-bristle brush, just like the one I have now. The heat from the hairdryer made the tips of my ears so red I thought they were burning. The process—taking sections of hair, chunk by chunk, and pulling them and rolling them and pulling them and rolling them—was as long and laborious as making homemade ravioli. But when it was done, oh lord. For the first time in my life, my hair was straight! Not board-straight, the way it might look if I got one of those Japanese hair-straightening treatments. Straight yet full of body, with that lovely underflip that I knew, the next day, would pull up and back to form the perfect ponytail I had always wanted but had never possessed.

When I got home that day, I worked at my computer for a while, but I didn't get much done. I was situated next to a mirror I had previously ignored, but suddenly I was swiveling in my chair to stare at myself, to make eyes at myself, to just *look*, with a pure happiness and confidence I had never experienced when looking into a mirror before. I know it is a stretch to say it was liberating. But things being what they are—in the way people look at themselves through the eyes of others, and in the way we size each other up in a glance, even if we wish and work to be above it and sometimes succeed—to sit there and look at myself and feel happy, it *was* liberating, indeed.

Except. Except! I felt liberated, and yet I had just been enslaved. Forget a scrunchy and an air-dry. I couldn't wash and go. It became impossible for me to be ready to do anything quickly post—hair washing, and the humidity that had always made my curly hair frizzy now threatened to undo and unravel my straight hairstyle at a moment's notice. I began bringing my own hairdryer everywhere, because most hotel hairdryers were not powerful enough to tame my curls. I felt like an idiot in front of my boyfriend (now husband) the first time we were forced to get ready together and I had to dry my hair in front of him, grimacing apologetically while he waited and waited for me to be ready to go, his stress mounting as the relentless drone of the hairdryer dragged on. He told me he would love my hair curly, but when I tried doing it that way, he was good enough to admit that he didn't really like the way it looked, either.

Aunt Patsy loved my blowout, of course. But my mother was dismayed by the change. As a straight-haired woman, she had never wavered in her conviction that my curls were a gift I should feel lucky to have been born with, and even at the height of my middle-school hair rage, she would actually say this to my face. If she was feeling particularly brave, she would go so far as to say, "Kamy, I would *kill* for your curls!" This really drove me nuts. For every straight-haired woman who has told a curly-headed woman, "I would kill for your curls," there is a curly-headed woman who would like to kill her for saying it. "You *think* you love my curls!" I used to want to scream, "but what you want are the curls you get when you have straight hair and somebody curls it!"

I remember once eyeing a woman with a beautiful head of long, wavy, romantically undulating hair in the salon where I get my hair cut in New York. My hairstylist, Fabrice—who cuts the hair of supermodels, actresses, and, most of the day, elderly society ladies who drive into Manhattan once a week from Scarsdale—caught my glance and immediately said, "Don't even look at her. Don't even look! Your hair cannot look like that. Those are waves. You have *curls*. Forget it! Banish it from your mind!"

Then he finished cutting my hair, gave me a kiss, turned to his assistant, and with a laughing look at me said, "Make it straight. She *loves* it straight."

Boy, was he right about that.

I blew my hair straight joyously for years. Twenty minutes a day and a little bit of humiliation and shame (and only in front of those who knew my secret—a small number, even after all these years) for twenty-four hours of hair happiness? No-brainer! But somewhere in the back of my mind, I always held on to the notion that this was a temporary state of affairs; that just as the blowout had come as a revelation to me, there was some way of styling my hair curly that would change my life with its effortless ease. I just hadn't heard about it yet. When I got pregnant, this vague hope acquired a greater sense of urgency. Didn't I need to simplify my life? To get my priorities straight?

At the time, I had a new friend who had become a very good friend, and she was a curly-haired friend too. I had never confessed my secret to her. There is no one I feel stupider in front of when I admit to the blowout than a woman with curly hair. Around these women I feel like a sellout, a poser, a coward, a cheat. But when I finally told Erin, in order to find out what *her* secret was (how did she have such lovely, cascading ringlets?), she reacted relatively kindly, with an amused, intrigued *"Reeeeaaaally?"* I'd heard before. Then she asked the unavoidable follow-up, delivered with curious but somewhat condescending nonchalance: "So what do you have to *do* to get it straight like that every morning?" This is akin to the question women who don't wear high heels ask women who do wear them, often pointedly and in front of accompanying men, "Are those *comfortable?*"—which is really a way of saying, "Are you really still so insecure that you are willing to be in pain while you walk just to impress men? How sad."

"What do *you* do to get your curls to look so great?" I countered. And as I asked, I felt the little spike of hope I'd felt a few times before when I'd told myself that finally, for real, I was going to stop the blow-drying and embrace my natural curl. Erin picked up on this immediately. I detected a familiar look in her eyes: the anticipation and excitement of a curly-haired woman who believed *she* would be the one to make me see the light. She uttered a single word—the name of a famous salon in New York specializing in curly hair—with a gravity and authority that hooked me immediately.

"This place changed my life," she averred. This did not seem like an overstatement to me. A hair salon totally devoted to curly-haired women!? I'd never heard of such a thing. I made an appointment for the next day.

It was November and chilly out when I walked into the salon the following afternoon. But as soon as I entered, I felt bathed in the warmth of a sea of gorgeous curls. The variations among the women there were endless, in skin color and every other way, but all of them were working their curls, and proudly. My heart beat a little faster. Clearly, I had arrived at Curl Mecca. And I was ready to be converted.

There was an evangelical feel to the place. Literature in the waiting area described the art of "training clients in the fundamentals of daily haircare and styling, encouraging and supporting them to embrace and enjoy their curls every day." Stylists were referred to as curl specialists, a.k.a. hydration specialists, "hydration being the key to happy, healthy curls." When my stylist beckoned, I smiled from ear to ear. Finally I would be *truly* free, with wash-and-go curls, just in time for my new life as a mom.

But it was not to be.

I spent three hours in that place. Three hours! First came what I expected: My hair was washed, then dried a bit, my curls were examined, and my hair was cut. It was what came next that killed me. "We are going to show you how to style your hair every day," my stylist told me. "It is very complicated to get curls right, and you must follow every step of this method exactly." Complicated? Method? My heart began to sink. And it only got worse. My marching orders: wash my hair with a product called Lo-Poo, which is not shampoo but something lighter that sort of kind of cleans your hair but, more important, does not weigh down your curls. Then stand, bend over, and turn your head upside down—gingerly shaking your hair out toward the floor—and slowly dab the excess water out of your hair with paper towels. (A real towel would be too harsh and interfere with the liberation of one's curls.) Continue standing in this position, even if the blood in your head is beginning to press heavily against the backs of your eyes, and scrunch two kinds of gel into your hair. (All products were available for sale at this salon, of course.) After that, take handfuls of tiny hair clips, twist small chunks of hair around your fingers until they look like tiny cinnamon buns, and clip them to your head so that they are lifted somewhat above your scalp. This will give your curls volume and height.

Talk about crazy! But, to be honest, I would have done it, or at least considered it as an alternative to sweating it out with my hairdryer. The curls that finally resulted from this process were wonderful, and it was the happiest I'd ever been with my curly hair. When all was said and done, I gravitated with fascinated pleasure toward every mirror I passed, seeing my curls look beautiful to me for perhaps the very first time. But there was just one problem: Even after all that scrunching and twirling and dabbing and gelling, the method wasn't done. After all that, you were allowed to touch your hair only once—to remove the clips at some point—and otherwise you were not supposed to touch it at all, ever, and you were supposed to let your hair dry in the air, for as many hours as that took. It was November. It was cold outside. I wanted dry hair, for Pete's sake! Was that so much to ask? Suddenly I remembered that any time before about 5:00 PM when I'd seen Erin, her hair had been wet. And I'd never, ever seen her touch it.

Frankly, I was pissed. The whole point of embracing my curls was supposed to be true freedom, ease! But at the same time, I felt validated. *Compared with this*, I thought, *the blowout is a real timesaver.* After all, one blowout lasts me not just one day but often two or three, as I can wake up in the morning with hair that is still semi-straight, smooth it out for a couple of minutes with my brush and my blowdryer (yes, I blow-dry my already dry hair), smear pomade all over it, and wear it in a ponytail that looks the way a ponytail is supposed to look . . . if you have straight hair. If I had curly hair, I would wake up with curly hair, except smashed by sleep-sweat. And then what? Do the method and air-dry? No thank you!

It was with no small amount of pleasure that I called Erin and asked, at last, the question my fellow curly-headed women were always asking me with such disdain.

"Do you seriously do this to your hair every day?"

She didn't flinch. "Yes," she said. "But not the paper towels. That's just dumb."

I know there are other ways to have curly hair. I know that I could let it dry in the air and it would look just fine, even lovely to some, but not to me. My best friend loves to let her hair air-dry in any sort of weather. But I don't. So what?

This would be a lovely place to conclude. A happy ending, or at least an ending: I am at peace with my addiction to the blowout! Many intelligent, secure, rational women—as I have long told myself—have at least one secret beauty-related idiocy they carry out in private—one time-consuming, silly thing they do in order to make looking in that inescapable mirror pleasant, or at least tolerable—and no one gets hurt. But this meditation would not be honest, or nearly as hilarious, if I did not confess a recent incident that called all of this logic severely into question in a whole new way.

After spending an afternoon working on this very essay, fifteen minutes before I was due to leave my apartment to participate in a panel discussion relating to my first book, I was transferring my hairdryer from one hand to the other—a move I have done a million times over the past thirteen years—and somehow I got it wrong. As the nozzle of the dryer swept past my face, the metal attachment that narrows the hot-air flow caught me in the eye. It was a severe, hot poke. I dropped the hairdryer with a jolt, jumped out of my seat, and covered my right eye with one hand. Tears poured down my face, and my eye felt as though a searing shish-kebab skewer had been thrust through it, as I paced around my apartment saying, "Oh no, no, no, don't do this, don't do this, don't do this," in no small part because of the utter embarrassment of having poked myself in the eye with my *hairdryer*. I prayed that it was just a temporary pain, a scratch, something that would feel better in moments so I could get on with my hair drying and my night.

But the pain didn't subside. It got worse. I called my husband, who was away with our sons (I was alone), and despite the mounting agony, I actually convinced myself that it would pass, that it was simply peaking, that I would be fine. And while I waited for that to happen, I sat back down in front of my mirror, examined the situation with my good eye, picked up my hair-dryer, *and finished drying my hair.*

There was only a little bit left to do. A few sections on the top. I wasn't sure if I was going to be okay, but I still hoped to participate in the panel, and if I did, I couldn't show up with three-quarters of my hair straight and one-quarter of it wet and scraggly!

I finished drying my hair, but I did not go to the reading. I went to the emergency room. I was fast-tracked (they don't screw around with eye stuff) and diagnosed with a conjunctival laceration and a corneal abrasion. It hurt so badly Vicodin didn't make a dent, and the only relief came when the nurse at the emergency room mercifully dropped numbing solution directly onto my eyeball. They told me that within twenty-four hours I'd feel a lot better, and that within a couple of days I would heal completely. Before leaving the emergency room, I had been forced to call the bookstore's events coordinator and tell her I'd be a no show because I had scratched my cornea with my hairdryer.

Do you think the universe was trying to tell me something?

I thought about this. I thought about this long and hard as I sat in my darkened apartment alone for two days, unable to watch TV or read, trying to find friends who would help me pass the hours either by talking to me on the phone or by coming over and chatting with me while I wore big, dark sunglasses. Erin, my curly-headed friend, just happened to be available, and telling her what had occurred made me feel incredibly dumb until I found out that she had just come from the curl salon, and that she had been there for hours and her hair was still wet. That brought a little smile to my face.

And Erin didn't make me feel bad. She didn't say, "So *now* are you going to stop this indefensible practice of pointing a red-hot sirocco at your head for twenty minutes, in danger of abrading your cornea or singing half the hair off your head, and come to your curly-girl senses?" Instead she said, "I'm loving the sunglasses indoors," and we talked for hours about other things. It was a nice moment between us, two curly-headed women who deal with it in different ways, two women who know that no matter how hard we may try to pretend it isn't true, and no matter how much we wish it weren't, we all have our thing when it comes to the way we look, and the blowout was mine, scratched cornea and all.

I am not at peace with my blowout. I am disheartened at the pleasure, confidence, and, yes, power I feel when I catch a glimpse of my hair in the mirror and I think it looks good. Everything about that is problematic if you think about it. Who says what looks good? Where do my ideas about that come from? Why is it so incredibly important for a woman to look good? Why has my husband never, not once, sat in the chair that I occupy so often in front of our vanity? What does the emphasis on a woman's looks mean about what she's for, and what she's worth?

At the same time, there is no denying that I am soothed and made happy by the pleasure, confidence, and empowerment I feel when I like my hair—as shaky as the foundation of those feelings may be. I am not twelve, but I am not immune to insecurity about my looks, either. And if I'm honest, I know that I will be making my hair straight for some time to come. (If a one-year-old boy, pulling on the cord and crying, "Mama!" doesn't deter me, what will?) Maybe I'm hopelessly vain. Or maybe it really is twenty minutes of silliness for twenty-four hours of a free pass from the anxiety I used to feel all the time about the way I looked. And maybe it's the reason that mirrors, at least for now, are no longer something for me to rage at or pray to. They are just something to put mascara on in front of—particularly useful if you wish to avoid poking yourself in the eye.

s. kirk walsh

RECONSTRUCTION: BEFORE & AFTER

When I look in the mirror, I often see the scars. There are many of them, collectively providing a barely visible topography of accidents, injuries, and surgeries that have occurred during my forty-one years of life. A small crescent-shaped scar punctuates my left eyebrow from a lager-fueled head-on collision during a friendly game of football in London's Hyde Park on Thanksgiving Day 1987. There is the scar that virtually serves as a second part in my hair from the removal of a benign cyst before I had the faculty of memory or language to recall the experience. A tiny half-moon indentation sits near my left ear, where a microsurgeon removed tissue in order to reconstruct the membrane of my eardrum, which had been perforated by multiple infections.

Then there are the other scars, the ones that you can't see. Most of them are inside my mouth, stretching along the interior of my gums and cheeks. With the tip of my index finger, I can feel the nubs of titanium wires just below the slick skin of my gums. When I was twenty-five years old, I underwent a daylong surgical procedure in which twenty-six wires and six ivy loops were used to wire my mouth shut. A titanium plate and multiple screws were also placed under the roof of my mouth to secure my upper jaw. I was hospitalized for five days and wired shut for seven weeks. Like any life-changing event, this surgery created a distinct *before* and *after*.

BEFORE

I sit with three other girls from my college in wicker chairs under a café's awning on the perimeter of the needle-shaped Piazza Navona in Rome. It is late October in 1986. Concerned about my expanding waistline due to nightly scoops of gelato, I order a plate of mozzarella, tomato, and basil leaves drizzled with balsamic vinegar. While I await my meal, I munch on pencil-size breadsticks and drink several glasses of white wine. Already, I am contemplating the glistening stainless steel troughs of brilliantly colored gelato at the nearby *gelateria*—and how I will refrain from ordering a *piccolo* while my friends indulge, again. At night, instead of recalling the magical interplay of shadows and light of Bernini's Four Rivers fountain in my journal, I write, "Watch out for that double chin!" I describe my face as "dumb, fat, and chubby."

A week later, I return to classes in London and make modifications to my daily routine: No breakfast except coffee with steamed milk. Attend crowded aerobics classes in the stale-smelling, subterranean studio of the Y, where I am living for the semester. Swear off red meat. Sugar—forget it! Then, on one particular night, my newfound regime takes on a disconcerting twist. When I stumble home late at night from the pub, after scarfing down a grease-stained paper container of chips, I discover the miracle of my index finger. All I have to do is reach it to the back of my throat—and just like that, the chips are hurling in the other direction. Just like that, the greasy potatoes are gone! Goodbye calories! Goodbye extra pounds!

After my semester abroad, I return to the isolated, snow-blanketed campus in upstate New York and live in a sorority with fifty other young women. On snowy Saturday afternoons, a group of us take to drinking shots of Jack Daniel's chased with swallows of Mad Dog. Eventually, we seek out lines of cocaine to extend the party into the night. I quickly discover that the fine white powder also acts as an appetite suppressant, taking the edge off my persistent hunger. When I return to the cold dorm, I lie awake in bed, listening to the shifting movements and breathing of the other young women as I slide my finger over the smooth edge of my protruding pelvic bone and the flatness of my stomach. This touch produces a tingling sensation that spirals to the center of my core. *This*, I think, *makes me pretty.*

I am twenty-four years old and living in New York City. With the help of others, I stop drinking. Not exactly what I had on the agenda for my mid-twenties, but this is what has happened. In an effort to refrain from drinking, I learn that eating three meals a day is a critical component of this new self-preservation equation. At first, I am not always aware of the fact that I'm hungry. Only when a friend asks me, "When is the last time you ate?" does it dawn on me that it's been more six than hours, and that eating something might be a good idea. Mostly, I eat in diners or get Chinese takeout. The only utensils in my kitchen are a can opener and a red-handled buck knife. During this time, I begin to notice men glancing in my direction. Though I still harbor concerns of a potential double chin, this criticism no longer serves as an ever-present chorus in the background of my mind.

Around the same time, I make the decision to undergo the jaw surgery. I have been aware of this possibility since I was sixteen years old, but promptly rejected the orthodontist's advice because I was just out of braces (the first attempt to correct my bite) and couldn't imagine going through the protracted ordeal that involved more metal in my mouth and seven weeks of being wired shut. Each time I go for another opinion, the doctors say the same thing as they hold the shadowy films of my misaligned teeth up to the illuminated lightboxes. *Your teeth don't hit. You don't chew food properly. Your digestion will be seriously compromised by the time you're forty.* In my mid-twenties, forty is the age of other, older people: my boss, who smokes cigars and reads Trollope novels. My oldest cousin, who regularly dyes her hair to camouflage its multiplying strands of gray. My gyne cologist, who has a framed picture of her two young daughters on her desk. This is what I consider instead of the fact that I can no longer bite into apples or chew red meat without leaving my jaw achy.

After five opinions, I listen to one doctor—Dr. M, a black-mustached man with a pair of tortoiseshell glasses and a lilting Indian accent. We are in his office on the eighteenth floor of the

Rockefeller Center, and he explains the complexity of the surgery to me for what feels like the tenth time. Heavy, wet snowflakes blow across the rectangular panes in the wrong direction. Below, crowds of tourists skate on the oval patch of ice, going round and round in circles, holding on to each other's waists, stretching the edges of their holiday sweaters. Prometheus—his thick arms outstretched with a ball of still-gold fire balanced in one hand—overlooks the circle of constant motion.

"Seven hours," Dr. M says, lightly moving his finger along the edge of his mustache, his voice soft and steady, "is the estimated length for the surgery."

Near the end of the appointment, he asks if there is anything else I would like to change. "Change?" I ask.

"While we're in there, we can make other changes to your face," he explains.

Abruptly, I say, "No, of course not!" I forget about the subtle protrusion of scar tissue on my lower lip from a lacrosse injury that sent me to the emergency room when I was a senior in high school. Instead, I think to myself that I'm just beginning to like my face, so why would I want to go and change it? Then Dr. M reminds me that there is one feature that will change, despite my reservations.

"You'll have more of a chin after the surgery," he explains, "because I'll be moving your lower jaw forward."

I nod, not saying a word. I come from a family of individuals who lack defined chins. During this moment, I don't consider this fact, nor Mr. M's comment. I'm more worried about the prospect of going under for six hours than I am about the profile of my postsurgery chin.

The next day, I'm having lunch with Michael at a coffee shop across the street from the music magazine where I work as an assistant editor. Cheeseburger for him. Grilled cheese for me. We split a plate of french fries with gravy. Michael and I have been friends for about ten months, having met at a writing workshop at the West 63rd Street Y. One of the first nights we went out, we saw a movie and then ate at a Greenwich Village institution known for its encyclopedic menu (almost nine hundred items) and surly cook/owner. Michael marveled at the selection, the possibilities. Midway through the meal, I walked into the bathroom and stared at my reflection in the mirror. My cheeks were flushed, my neck an uneven patchwork of crimson. I talked to my reflection, wondering if this was possible. *I like him, a lot.*

About six months later, I visit Michael on the set of his latest film in Bluefield, West Virginia. He has been cast in the starring role of a white supremacist, who returns to his hometown to try to force his parents' marriage back together. From the onset, our visit feels off. Michael drives recklessly on the winding backcountry roads. The long-lashed actress playing opposite him is clearly interested in him. At night I cry myself to sleep, knowing that I never should have come. Now, sitting across from each other in the coffee-shop booth, I still long for something more than friendship, but deep down, I know that it's unlikely.

That night on the phone, after our lunch, I pose the inevitable question to Michael: "Is there a future in this relationship for you?" After a protracted silence, he says no. The edges of my heart ache. I haven't liked anyone the way I like Michael in some time. I like the sweetness of his smile. I like how I can be around him and not worry about what I'm wearing. Sometimes I even feel pretty. I try to recall the unpleasant parts of our story—the visit to West Virginia, Michael's moodiness.

"I don't think I can see you for a while," I struggle to say. A tear slides into the crease of my nose as I hold the receiver against my hot ear. After a few more words, he says goodbye, pauses, and says, "Good luck with the surgery."

The day before the surgery, I'm admitted to Columbia Presbyterian at 168th Street and Broadway. The following morning I wake at six o'clock to a rush of people moving around me. I am a stone in the middle of a stream, the water pushing in all directions.

"Let's get her going," one of the orderlies says.

I want to say, "Wait. No. I'm not ready."

Two orderlies wheel a gurney next to my bed and lift me onto it. They tuck a white sheet over my body. I look up at the ceiling. Long, narrow tubes of fluorescent lights pass over me in a blur. They wheel me into a waiting room of gurneys. I can't see anyone's face (I am almost blind without my contact lenses or glasses). A warm voice approaches me. It's my anesthesiologist, Dr. W. His round beige face appears before mine. I can see his white teeth.

"You're going to be okay," he says, lightly touching my arm. Next thing I know, someone is pushing my gurney into a bright white room. The familiar voice of Bob Seger sings. *Against the wind. We'll be running, running against the wind.* One of the nurses sings along softly, arranging the shiny instruments on a nearby cart. My body relaxes as Dr. W sticks a long needle into the bend of my arm.

"Breathe," he says. "Breathe."

AFTER

I have been in the hospital for five days now, and Dr. M strongly suggests that I leave. I want to trust his brown eyes, but I find this hard to believe: I can't imagine getting by without the IV, the oxygen. I can barely sip a cup of water, let alone ingest two thousand liquid calories a day—what Dr. M says I need to heal properly. He pats me on the knee and tells me that it's going to be okay. He reminds me that the operation was only inside my mouth; everything else inside my body is working just fine. Dr. M tells me to get dressed and that the nurse will be by momentarily to discharge me.

Since the surgery, I haven't looked at my face in the mirror. Mom tells me not to. She says that with my swollen, puffed-up cheeks, I look like Dizzy Gillespie blowing his horn. Dr. M says it will take at least a month for my face to return to its former size.

Before the surgery, it was decided that my own apartment—a three-flight walkup, no bathtub, and tons of street noise from Avenue A infiltrating the thin tenement walls—wasn't the ideal location for my two-week recovery. Instead, I will stay in a room at the Excelsior Hotel on West 81st Street, across from the Museum of Natural History. Mom will stay with me for the first week, and then my older sister will stay for the second week. When a nurse wheels me to the hospital's front entrance, a cab awaits Mom and me in the circular drive. After we are settled in the car, Mom reminds the driver that I have just had surgery, to drive slowly with no abrupt stops or turns. He nods and starts driving. I'm still wondering if I can do this— begin to heal without the liquid IV sustenance, the cool inhalations of oxygen, the around-the-clock care. Hanging from the oversize rearview mirror are strands of colorful plastic beads and a playing card–size image of Jesus Christ—his hand held in front of him, a nimbus glowing around his head. Every time the car goes over a pothole, my jaw aches. The beads jangle. Jesus swings from side to side. All I can see are my eyes and forehead in the driver's rearview mirror.

My days are focused on one objective: drinking enough calories to heal. In the hospital, I lost nine pounds, and Dr. M says I need to gain it back. In order to accomplish this, I drink multiple cans of Ensure (chocolate and vanilla), usually up to six per day. We try milkshakes with bananas, but even the tiny black seeds in the bananas get caught in between the wires. Watered-down baby food (carrots and peas) doesn't work out so well either, so I stick to Ensure. During the first week, I rarely crave solid foods. Instead, I am amazed by the early milestones of my recovery—taking a bath, walking a half block with Mom on one side of me, sitting on a bench in the nearby park to watch the squirrels dance from branch to branch, being able to read again. Sleeping through the night proves to be more difficult. I wake up from nightmares, my arm caught in a phantom tangle of plastic tubing. When I open my eyes, all I see are the fading black-and-blue marks in the bends of my arms.

During these sleepless nights, I find myself thinking of Michael, often. He lives only five blocks south of the hotel. I wonder what he is doing right now. Is he still in New Mexico for the holidays? Eventually, I drift back to sleep as the barks of dogs float up to the hotel's eleventh floor.

Getting around the city of New York with a wired jaw proves to be an interesting challenge. I carry a notepad, a pen, and a pair of pliers at all times. (Dr. M explained several times that pliers were more of a psychological measure, so I knew that I had the means to clip my mouth open at any second.) Most people, strangers, speak to me as if I am mute. Many of them end up yelling at me, even though I can hear perfectly fine. I continue on my daily diet of Ensures. I blend milkshakes with Häagen-Dazs, eggs, and Hershey's syrup. I buy pints of warm chicken broth from the Second Avenue Deli. I steadily gain back the nine pounds.

When I return to work, there are multiple one-way conversations with coworkers curious about my wired condition. I'm ever prepared, with my battery of answers written down on a folded piece of yellow legal paper: "I had jaw surgery. I will be wired shut for three more weeks. I'm feeling much better. It was for medical reasons. My teeth didn't hit right. Thanks."

One such conversation is with the magazine's photo editor. As we leave the office kitchen, she comments, "That must be a great way to lose weight." A knot of anger twists up in my stomach. I don't even begin to try to explain that this has nothing to do with losing weight. It would require too much writing.

The unwiring of my jaw is an anticlimactic event. First of all, it hurts much more than I thought it would. I am mildly sedated on nitrous oxide before Dr. M clips and then yanks the wires from my gums. Drops of blood splatter the paper sheet hanging from the clipped chain around my neck. After he is done, I can barely open my mouth, because the muscles have atrophied during the past six weeks. When it comes time for my first meal, I go to a café on 18th Street and 8th Avenue with two friends and order a side of mashed potatoes and gravy. I eat four bites before giving up. It's too hard to open my mouth wide enough for the fork. Instead, I go home and drink another Ensure.

A month later, Michael and I run into each at the movies. I knew he was in the theater before I even saw him, because I heard his familiar laugh amid the sold-out audience. We make small talk in the popcorn-pungent lobby while my friends wait near the door. Michael asks if he can call me. Later, to my amazement, he invites me over for dinner. He makes a simple meal of tortellini with sautéed onions, garlic, mushrooms, and basil. A tossed salad with mustard vinaigrette. I sit nervously at the table in his living room. He fills two water glasses with seltzer, the effervescent bubbles grabbing at the smooth sides. Curls of steam rise from the generous plates of pasta. Michael clinks his glass against mine—and we eat. Later, he would tell me that something was different about my face when we ran into each other at the movie theater that night.

"My chin?" I ask.

"That," he says, "and something else." During my recovery, the swollenness has slowly subsided and my old face has begun to take shape. Michael is not the only person to have noticed a change, but it is something that I can't see.

That spring, Michael and I begin to play tennis at the courts in Central Park on a biweekly basis. He invites me to his apartment to watch a television show where he plays the guest star (a petty criminal who helps to infiltrate the Ku Klux Klan in the rural South). I say no. I'm hesitant. I don't want to get hurt again. Eventually, he asks me out on an official date. I say yes, somewhat reluctantly. We meet at the Guggenheim Museum for

an exhibition of iron sculptures by artists such as Alberto Gia-
cometti, Pablo Picasso, and David Smith—fluent pieces of metal
bent into organic shapes that are equal parts whimsical and
provocative. We start at the top of the spiral, and as we wind our
way down the circular pathway, our body language begins to
shift. Michael touches me against the small of my back; his fin-
gertips lightly graze my arm. By the spiral's bottom, he threads
his fingers between mine. And at the end of our date, he gives
me a kiss on the lips before we go our separate ways—and it feels
like something electric.

Once we begin to date seriously, I ask Michael why he
changed his mind about me. He refers to the surgery, how my
face has more definition. He says that I'm more of a classic
beauty. I wonder if this is a good thing.

What's with this guy? I think. *Is this the kind of person I
want to be with?*

Later, when I press Michael further, it is evident that other
changes have taken place in his life. Soon I learn that he was ingesting handfuls of barbiturates on a regular basis while he was
working on the film in West Virginia. He has maintained an er-
ratic, self-destructive relationship with drugs and alcohol since
he was a young child (he was raised on communes, where pot
and tabs of acid were readily available). It has been six months
since Michael has taken a drug or drink. He continues to say
that it's my face, but I begin to think it's his perception.

In hindsight, it is a difficult exercise to pinpoint the exact
cause and effect of the surgery. I do know this much: Before the
surgery and before this relationship with Michael, I never felt
beautiful. I was a relentless critic of my own appearance. Never

pretty enough. Never thin enough. After the surgery and after my ongoing relationship with Michael (we've been married ten years now), I can recognize why others might be attracted to me. Indeed, it helps that Michael tells me that I'm beautiful all the time—and the great thing is, I actually believe him.

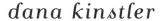

dana kinstler

THE PUNK
INFANTA

On my pillow. My father left the pencil drawing of Richard Nixon on my white pillowcase, where I found it one night as I stumbled in from a nightclub. I was startled at the familiar visage in strong profile, Nixon's mouth pulled back in a quick smile. Beneath his head, this note: "Dear D., Sweet Dreams! Love, Richard."

I snorted, removing my tight black jeans and ripped and safety-pinned T-shirt. I know his faux inscription, dated January 1980; he's playing Tricky Dick. I admired the depiction, one I knew my father did in less than three minutes—he'd captured the classy brow and the way even a liar's smile has sincerity in the corners of the mouth.

My father is in the face business—not cosmetics or plastic surgery, but portraiture: faces stuck in time, glued in with pigment on gesso-covered canvases, faces made permanent, lives transcendent, hanging forever on a wall. Inside my childhood apartment, faces were everywhere. Faces on the kitchen wall looked down at us over our dinner plates—actresses, presidents, corporate executives, my sister, my mother, Elvis Presley, all painted in the same style: floating heads on half torsos, smiling, looking their best, oftentimes presented from the side. These were my father's portraits, ones he painted for a living, faces I felt closer to, sometimes, than I did to my own. The portrait of me was a watercolor, zoomed in, at age three, exuberant, chin dimple emphasized, smile in my hazel eyes.

That watercolor was always how I saw myself. But by age seventeen, my perception of that portrait started to change. Sitting below it, consciously *not* eating dinner, I found my own image alienating. I couldn't study it too long; it cast an eerie shadow, as if I were looking into a dead girl's face, three-year-old gone to an early grave. Scrutinzing my portrait, I was reminded of headstones upstate, dark gray slabs carved with angel wings hanging over the etched dates of a child's life. At seventeen, I had the peculiar sense that having been painted, I was dead. I knew instinctively that the point of the portrait was to preserve life as you had it *at this moment*; soon after, you may as well have croaked, since your face would be forever saved in the wooden frame. Paintings last longer than the person. That's the point.

My family went to one art museum only; we took outings to the Metropolitan Museum of Art. I'd been going since I was a baby, carried by my parents up the steps to this temple of high art. Inside, oil paintings and marble sculptures made me feel alive.

Each pope, baby Jesus, Madonna, Mercury, Athena—each with their own wild headgear: miter hat, veil, or wreath—was of another time. I knew I wouldn't run into any Christian icons or Grecian gods when I left the museum and walked back into the Lexington Avenue subway (although during summer or Halloween, the lower downtown I got, I passed their lookalikes vamping and stomping near Washington Square Park).

As a teenager, I ran through the galleries alone, but always on a singular quest: I wanted to study the portraits. The Spanish *infantas*—baby queens—painted with lap dogs at their ankles, in white lace collars, wearing rings, jeweled shoes, already holding the weight of their empires in their brows; why else wear white doilies in the morning? Dutch faces were dour, had landscapes outside their windows, children trapped indoors; the French wore frilly dresses and stockings; British children were coupled with hounds whose mouths were soft with the broken necks of dead pheasants, girls and boys wistful in their pale luminescence. Their faces were full of longing—for careless play, for a fleeting liberty—and so composed as to appear dignified, but paint had fixed their expressions. Their faces revealed the burden of sovereignty, of too much wisdom, their large, round eyes glowing beneath high foreheads. I knew they were painted not barefoot in a sunny patch of woods, chasing a liver-spotted setter, but actually standing stiff in a curtained room indoors. *Stay perfectly still! Quit the twitching!*

I often wondered if the portraits' subjects had wanted to cease the posturing, stand up, and bolt. If you were sitting for a portrait, you were, in essence, captured, kept in your role—as royal personage, as hero, as martyr, as slave.

On his love seat. Once, my father spontaneously painted an oil sketch, entitled *With Thumb and Blanky*, while I lay on my side, Manet-style, pink blanket caressing my cheek, hazel eyes the luminous focal points on the canvas, legs crossed in white tights, brown school shoes dangling toward an empty space. The only parameter of my body was his love seat; his brushstrokes were few, paint thinned with turpentine; beneath me, the ground disappeared into a limbo of middle earth, as if only the sky held me up. Set in this netherworld of paint-time, in custody of my father's aura, being painted seemed to stop minutes, carve me out a space, alone in his studio, lying still, waiting for his gaze, absorbed in an adoration that could come only spontaneously, his hands motivated by something I could not comprehend. We were uninterrupted, something that occurred only when my sister and mother were not in the room, precious flickering moments, and then it didn't matter what I looked like at all. There was a freedom in time distorted while posing. Upon completion, I was pleased. Although out of focus, it felt like me. I was comfortable as a sketch.

I knew what it felt like to not see myself at all. You could never comprehend the artist's portrait: your face through the prism of their vision, their hands, their painting style; their love or dislike or even fear of you. An artist can't paint you if they're not captivated; the artist's hand responds to an insistence as fierce as the itch of poison ivy. *It had to mean something*, I'd always thought as a girl. Even if you'd commissioned the portrait yourself, still, there's attachment. It wasn't just about dollars and cents—you craved to view how you were seen.

Along the long hallway. It shot out of my dad's studio, then curved and split—this way to my room, which I shared with my older sister; that way to my parents' bedroom. It was lined with more paintings, early pen-and-ink illustrations, pulp-fiction jacket covers, and comic strips. There were charcoal sketches and oil portraits of my mother, her pale hair piled high, her sharp blue eyes looking into a distance over our heads and beyond. Her profile with upturned nose, her ample chest. Intermingled with these were nude women whose breasts I didn't recognize, women sprawled open, leaning back in chairs, one naked in our own kitchen. One had nipples the size of John F. Kennedy half-dollars, another's were more like bright copper pennies. These pictures were our extended clan.

Before my sister or I was born, my father had inked pictures for bodice rippers and comic strips. I passed them en route to my bedroom: cowboys rescuing barmaids whose lace-up blouses had come undone, rodeo bulls bucking in the background, lassos circling overhead. Space captains snatching up extragalactic princesses, freeing them from the one-eyed bubble-headed, encephalitic Martians, space guns shooting their mile-long interminable rays in the dark sky. Doctors holding buxom, doe-eyed, swooning nurses; sheriffs grasping wavy-haired cowgirls; men in masks freeing women just busting from their bikini tops, holding evil predators at bay. These duos rode away into the hills or flew on spaceships toward Earth, but always, the females were rescued.

As a girl, I'd been enthralled, seen my father as captor and hero both, a magnificent force who drew magic scenarios and could dump the inkwell on them if he wanted. I'd studied where the nib of his fountain pen pooled, where it zipped up into a curlicue, where he'd used furious cross-hatching to separate the background from a face, where just a line—my father's hand dragging up and across the paper like a swashbuckler slashing open a bandit's neck—had become the visceral focal point on the page. Yet I could not see me in these drawings. I searched but never found myself—the girl with hazel eyes, freckles, and glasses—getting rescued by the hunk savior. I assumed less pretty females like me stayed on the alien planet with the Martians or lived among the outlaws. That's where I worried I'd find myself if I could live inside one of my father's illustrations, which was what I wanted to do.

I had an asymmetrical face: one eye higher than the other, a long nose, a freckle-dappled forehead and widow's peak. None of the pen-and-ink females had freckles. As a teenager, passing this wall in order to reach my own room, I reacted to a line, an illustrative gesture, a character's remark. I'd once seen them as my inky fairies who watched over me from behind glass on the wall, but now I took offense at these females. Their breasts spilling out of their blouses and cone-style brassieres, and their kitten-seductive eyes and pursed lips, now bore a passivity that enraged me. Their mouths were painted shut, faces in motionless adoration, beneath the heroes, faces without dialogue captions. Voluptuaries need not speak.

I knew the cosmic-dialogue quips, uttered them by rote in my nasal deadpan, without a glance, en route to my room: "Deep in the canyon, by the Ranch L-Bar-Horseshoe, the outlaws have tied up Miss Betty Sue to the lone cactus!" ran the editorial hanging on the upper left-hand corner like a first-page prologue, providing necessary tension. "I'll Save You, Princess! Zap! Hands off, brute!" I'd smooch out a long embrace: *Pssxx slurp!*

Now I'd fill in, "Return me C.O.D. to my Martian, slugg-o thug-o! At least get some cool jeans!"

When a potential suitor came over to take me out, I'd make sure to nonchalantly drag him back past the picture wall—as if it were a final checkpoint before entering my room. Would he turn away upon viewing these sexy idols with button noses and uncontainable breasts? What if one of the bombshells reached out and grabbed him by the collar, offering herself in exchange for my unexotic self?

"Whoa! So cool!" That was the usual response. It was as if the space-gun rays had zapped his mind, reducing his response to monosyllables. This boy, my secret favorite, was my neighbor. He glanced at my watercolor, then stopped in his tracks. These: our nudes. The fall of one's breast, the opening of another one's legs, sunlight glancing off her upturned nipples, then dappling her pale thighs.

"Your dad painted her in your kitchen?"

I watched him lick his lips. Indeed, our kitchen—with faux-brick linoleum floors, round plastic-coated table, light streaming through hanging spider plants that rested in my mother's homemade macramé holders. I'd never dared to ask exactly when this sitting had taken place; I had always waited for my mother's cues. Suddenly my companion had an entire relationship with these nudes, which undoubtedly accompanied him as he made his way into my bedroom.

In his camera. Like a painting that pulls together technique, subject, light, all presenting in that right moment—like Manet's *Le Déjeuner sur l'herbe*—varying elements came together the spring of my seventeenth year. It was the end of the 1970s; I was about to graduate from high school, I had my first boyfriend, and I longed to be set free from the ideals of my household. Several nights a week we stepped out to Max's Kansas City, a neighborhood club. And that May, my father painted Miss America.

She appeared that spring, and subsequent springs, newly elected, on tour, contest winner, gown on a hanger, tiara on a pillow, chaperone waiting in my dad's studio; as he prepared his palate, Miss America scurried into our bathroom to change into her gown.

She left her day clothes—red-skirted suit, cream silk blouse, and nylon day panties—on a hook where my mother hung her terry robe.

My father snapped copious photos during that one visit, which he'd use to paint her portrait, and I snuck in to study them, finding nothing irregular, nothing to shatter her balanced, china-doll features—eyes and nose neither too small nor too large—all in proportion, a perfect example of flawless beauty, like you'd see on a marble sculpture at the Met.

Later, over dinner, I grilled my dad: Had she offered her view on U.S. involvement in Latin America, for instance? Did she know how we had financed all the worst dictators in history? Was her chaperone just a matron, stationed to humiliate and downstage the crowned beauty like a big, homely baby sitter? Did the chaperone turn on some Shirley Temple tune and get the Miss to tap-dance in his studio? I baited, attempting to engage him in my diatribe about her false demeanor—made-up eyes, Laura Petrie hair, fakey-fake smile. My mother sighed, serving the green beans, as he and I went at it.

During this period, I made a new friend who was an abstract artist and a daughter to filmmakers; she smuggled me into uptown museums to expose me to modern art, shocked at my ignorance. I'd never had the daring to visit any of the hipper museums that exhibited living artists. Uptown with her, I began to see myself inside a cubist painting, my patchwork innards externalized; here were artists who sold art based on a disjointed interior, the fragmented self restitched together. Or not. I found a place for my disheveled self. Some forms of art—primitive, emotive—felt childlike, and something internal began to shift.

The art of my father, portrait art, stirred in me a secret passion for what rebelled against it—free shapes, whimsy, meaningless swatches of color; Matisse, Picasso, Miró; and yet I noticed I was still drawn to individuals, to modern portraits in one form or another.

I'd have painted Chrissie Hynde, Lydia Lunch, Tina Weymouth: the women I saw onstage, some with hair down around their faces, bangs hiding their eyebrows, sometimes even their eyes; they moved with a swagger, a chord, punctuating with the sudden blast of amp feedback; they held beer cans, slung guitars over their shoulders. Eye makeup and lipstick always; buns and lacy neck pieces never. They reigned, their energy as tight and electrifying as the sound of a switchblade snapping open; they might have been caught hanging around outlaws who slashed a painting in an uptown gallery in the middle of the night, then polluted the subway tunnel with spray paint all the way up and off the white tiles.

I was captivated by women with spiked dyed hair, in fishnets, vinyl skirts, ripped T-shirts, and black leather jackets. And bangs. None of the females in my Dad's portraits had bangs.

Back in our apartment, I retrieved the scissors from my dad's desk and handed them to my friend. When she raised the pair of scissors to my wavy, reddish-brown hair and made the first cut, I was sure my father could hear the incision down the hall.

"Bangs!" my father shouted. "You ruined your face!" It was as if I'd punched him.

"Everyone has bangs!" I rolled my eyes, a new tic, avoiding his gaze.

For my high school graduation, I hennaed my hair Vermillion Red Light, bought a vintage Light Magenta gown with a beaded neck, and put on Brilliant Rose pumps, ignoring my father's sneers about clashing hues and about how unattractive it was when women hid their foreheads. I was Rita Hayworth. My boyfriend commented that my eyeliner and mascara were good, as they cleared up the general "mishmash" of my face.

By the time Miss America stopped coming, I was already gone—off to college in New England. But every spring I recalled her arrival—just after school, amid the warm light in the park where the tulips sprang up in explosive display. How I watched for her limousine, crouching in the park with my former boyfriend. As the limo door opened, he stood and belted out, "Here she comes . . . Miss America . . . " much to my horror and shame. It was one thing to poke fun of her at home, another to do it in public.

But something else: If the portrait was a person—I'd hear a voice in the hall, anticipate a sitter's appearance—an apparition fleshed out, an image already known from a sketch or photo or thin layer of paint—as the voice moved closer, I tracked it like a deepwater creature using echolocation, wanting to hide.

If I heard laughter, knew my father was telling one of his long, intricate jokes, I could have knocked on the door if I'd wanted; I would have seen her, any of the women whose oil sketches I'd lived with for the past few months—but I didn't want to be disappointed in what I'd find. If we met, I'd mumble hello, make eye contact, smell her breath, find a crumb on her lip, notice eye makeup smeared—mascara clumped on a lash, roots seeping in behind blond locks. The nose and eyes were never what they were in oil paint; I preferred what remained on the wall, because inside each frame were a mystery and a familiarity, a piece of myself, parts of someone else. What would she say if she could speak? Most likely, I'd never know, but I craved the knowledge, and this *not knowing*, but *imagining*, was vital. What I liked to do was study the way my father dabbed points and globs of paint to create a crown that sparkled more on canvas than it did in real life.

My father and I sit without talking in a Boston hotel lounge, sipping late-afternoon coffee, smoking cigarettes. I've ridden the bus up from college in Providence to visit him, where he's on a commission. Outside, the Boston Common shimmers with the life of city ponds—swans, bronze ducklings, pigeon crap, the homeless asleep on benches. My father picks up a pen from inside his jacket, then sketches my profile as I gaze out over the park. We are quiet, and in this silence there is both trust and discomfort, the kind I welcome—it is not easy to be a gracious sitter after all these years. When he finishes, I am amazed—who is this female, her nose from the side, wispy forehead bangs, the strength in her jawline? He has captured me, captured something of the determination and wisdom I've been told are my salient qualities; in that profile, I see something I haven't before: his *respect*, like that which he gave to Richard Nixon and Miss America. He is viewing me through an artist's eyes, passionate, detached, doing what he must—sketching the picture because my nose perhaps interested him a little too much, or my brow presented a challenge. Here is my father, and here, as an adult, I have walked away from the firing range at last and am capable of simply offering him my best profile.

catherine texier

SELF-PORTRAIT WITH MIRROR

My mother was stricken by a cerebral hemorrhage a few years ago in the South of France, where she lived part of the year. I sat by her side at the hospital in shock and dismay, along with one of my uncles. By the time I had gone to the Nice airport to pick up my daughters, who were flying from New York, she had passed away. She had already been taken to the morgue when we pulled into the parking lot. The girls couldn't bear to see their nanny dead, and so I went to the mortuary alone and sat on a bench, waiting. A man came shuffling through a back door after a while and asked: You're coming to see your mom?

Yes, I said.

He looked at me for a moment and said gently: There's nothing to be scared about. It's just your mom.

He disappeared through a back door and returned a few moments later, pushing a gurney covered with a white sheet.

I stood up stiffly, my heart beating.

He looked at me with compassion.

Come, he said.

He walked me to the gurney and pulled the sheet off her face.

Her skin was pulled taut, shrunken over her bones, the cheekbones prominent, the forehead high, the whole face sculpted as if in stone. She didn't look that different from the way she had looked that morning when I had left her, her forehead banded with a furrow from the respirator they had fitted her with to help her breathe.

You can kiss her, the man said in a soothing voice. There's nothing to fear.

I leaned forward and brushed her forehead with my lips, where the respirator had left the red mark, and that's when I knew for sure that she was gone, her spirit flown away.

Her face felt taut and dense, like a plaster cast. All her life stuffed into that rigid cast with no room to move, no room to add anything.

The face reduced to its bone structure. To its architecture.

I thought: *This was my grandmother's face when I saw her wrapped in the traditional Vendée white shroud. This will be my face too when I die.*

I've always looked like my mother, but for a long time I didn't know it. Others saw it, but I didn't. It took years for life to chisel the cheekbones, to sharpen the roundness of the cheeks and the chin, for the eyes to gaze straight or playfully, instead of hiding under a veil of shyness. And it took years for me to accept my mother's inheritance. Now, when I catch my face in the mirror, especially an accidental glimpse in a street window, a random glance in a bathroom mirror, I see her. It startles me, because it's not so much a resemblance as a reincarnation. It's not just that the features are remarkably similar—except for my nose, which is rounder at the tip, not perfectly and delicately straight like hers was. It's as if her expression, her smile, the seductive glint in her eyes, have been breathed into me. With a shock, I realize that I have finally let her spirit live in me instead of repressing it deep inside.

Because of her violent scenes, her provocations, her communist beliefs, her disappearances, her chaotic affairs, her irresponsibility, my mother was constantly put down by my grandparents. They offered to take care of me when she got pregnant by accident with a man who wouldn't marry her, and we lived with them until I was fourteen and she moved away. Growing up, I existed in a state of terror at expressing any "forbidden" emotion, which was any emotion (rage, anger, passion, excitement) that might be associated with her, and you can tell, looking at photos taken during my childhood and teenage years, that my face was frozen stiff. Photos taken when I was older show a startlingly different face: sensual, flirtatious, and open, where it used to be guarded and closed in. It is the face I've kept since my late twenties and thirties, in spite of the frown lines that have appeared between the eyebrows, the creases that now trace a line between the nose and the corners of the mouth, and a softening of the jawline.

My resemblance to my mother appeared gradually, like a negative slowly exposed in a fixing bath. It revealed itself more and more as I traveled farther and farther away from her, as if the distance, both geographical and emotional, allowed our resemblance to assert itself. And beyond the resemblance to my mother, I can see the cheekbones and the round cut of my grandmother's face, the face of a young girl from Vendée, a French province on the Atlantic coast. And past her, like overlapping watermarks or an infinite perspective of mirrors, emerge the faces of my grandmother's sister and her nieces, my great-grandmother who taught elementary school in a little seaside village in the early part of the twentieth century, and my other great-grandmother, the school principal and healer. Generations of Vendée women with the same cheekbones and the same green or hazel eyes, whom I imagine—going back two or three centuries, way before the revolution—toiling as artisans' wives or chambermaids in the castles of noblewomen. Comely, shapely maidens fit to play pretty chambermaids in a Molière play, or perhaps the lead *jeune première* role in a Racine drama. In spite of an underlying stubbornness, our faces evoke those French words: *accorte, avenante, gracieuse*—spry, spunky, vivacious, graceful. I know that I'm not destined to turn into a matron, as my mother never did, even at eighty-five, when she died, nor did her mother before her, who passed away at ninety-seven. Somehow, the girlishness doesn't go away.

I was already in my forties when I first met my father. I had finally summoned the courage to ask my mother if she had any idea where he was. She thought he still lived in Villefranche-sur-Mer, near Nice, on the Côte d'Azur. I found his address by calling the phone company. I sent him a letter, and he wrote me back, and we agreed to meet in a little village in the hills between Nice and Grasse in Provence. An older man with a shock of white hair and an aquiline nose, he looked nothing like me. At the end of lunch, when he showed me pictures of his children and grandchildren, I stared at them avidly.

There they were, my half sister and half brothers, with their respective husbands or wives and children, and none of them looked like me at all. But you can't always trust pictures, so I asked him if he saw any resemblance. He said no. Then I asked him if he saw a likeness between him and me.

He looked at me pensively and shook his head.

No, he did not.

Suddenly it mattered very much to me to look like him or like his children, maybe because it was so abstract otherwise, sitting next to this man whom I had never met before in my life. How could I even be sure that he was my father? What if my mother had slept with a different man around the same time? The idea flashed through my mind, lingered for a moment, and faded. There had been enough drama in my childhood; I didn't need to create more out of my fantasy. When I went back to my mother's house later that day, I sat in front of the mirror and tilted my head up and down and at an angle, and thought I recognized something in the space between my nose and my lips that made me think of him. But the resemblance was elusive, a flutter, a mirage, as if for an instant his spirit had entered me, and a moment later my features had reassembled themselves and I couldn't capture him anymore.

There's hardly any trace of my father in my face. At least, hardly any trace that I can see. Since I didn't grow up with him,

I didn't pick up his expressions, the way a child unconsciously mimics her parents. Maybe I am just not familiar enough with his face. Or maybe I just look more like my mother.

When I first moved to New York, I shared an apartment with a Turkish friend who used to say, "I have to put my face on" every morning when she got up. Maybe it was a translation from the Turkish, but I think she meant more than the application of foundation and eye shadow on her bare skin. Applying make-up, for her, equated "face," or made-up mask. She didn't have a "face" until she had prepared it to "face" the outside world.

When I wake up in the morning, I too feel that my face is a blank canvas, which I have to prepare to "face" life. And I don't mean makeup, which I wear very little of anyway. Rather, it's that the night seems to wash away the previous day's expressions, like the gray sky of dawn, before it comes alive with the interplay of sun and clouds. So, too, my face is a changing sky of moods. Face in repose: waiting to be filled with emotions, expressions, inner fire. Face after love: brimming with pleasure. Seductive face: a brilliant smile. Passionate face: flushed, vibrant, open, with shiny eyes. Depressed face: pinched, inert, drained with fatigue, fear. Blank, unmade-up face in the morning while I am about to sit down at my computer to write, while still in my pajamas, harks back to the plainness of village life in Vendée. High energy and vibrant face, with a little makeup before going out, evokes my mother's seductiveness and life force.

You're pretty, they said, when I was finally able to hear compliments without doubting them. I still hear them. I tally the good features: the bone structure. The cut of the face. The cheek-bones and the jawline. The point of the chin. A certain harmony in the lines. The mouth, delicately drawn. The curve of the eye-brows, still well shaped. For a long time I thought the space be-tween the nose and the mouth was a bit too long. Ironically, that is precisely the feature I now think comes from my father—it's my least favorite one, even as I try to see his face in my own. When I met one of my half brothers, I noticed his nose was a bit bulbous at the end, and I wondered if the tip of my nose might have been inherited from a distant grandmother or grandfather on my father's side, in Auvergne, the heart of France.

The eyes. It's vain, no doubt, to admit it, but I like my eyes. They are large, and hazel–green, and I draw the inside of the lids with dark kohl like a Maghrebian woman. When I am in Paris I buy real kohl in the Moroccan shop at the big mosque. It's a pow-derlike substance of dark bluish–gray, which is applied with a narrow wooden stick. Its subtle glitter deepens the gaze, making it sultry and sexy. Otherwise I use a black kohl pencil. When I discovered, around the age of twelve, that I had to sit in the first row in math class in order to read the equations on the black-board, and the ophthalmologist confirmed that I had to wear glasses, I collapsed in sobs. My life was doomed, or at least my fu-ture as a potentially attractive girl was. I had no idea yet whether I was an attractive girl or not, but the hideous glasses shot down all hope of my ever becoming one. Sometime in my late teens, though, boosted by my own observations and the way boys hit on me, I decided to be an attractive girl, with or without glasses.

I would have loved to wear contact lenses, but my eyes are too dry to wear them comfortably, so the glasses—like my hair, later—became a prop, an accessory that I turned to my advantage. In the '70s, I wore wire-rimmed granny glasses when they were all the rage. With my loose, curly hair, they gave me a hippie look. When I met my ex-husband, who is even more myopic than I, we were both wearing old-fashioned, round, tortoiseshell frames. I loved that our styles matched—*a couple of cool writers with glasses*, I thought, *we are meant to be together!* Nowadays I wear plastic-framed glasses, in a trendy rectangular shape, which make me feel like a sexy nerd.

It took me longer to accept my tightly curly hair, which my grandmother would braid in two tresses every morning before school, after epic brushing sessions. For a few years, I straightened it using various barbaric techniques, flattening it wet around my skull in overlapping, concentric layers, then covering it with a scarf and sleeping on it, or wrapping it over huge rollers and blow-drying it straight (that was before the Japanese or Brazilian methods, and before the flattening iron was invented). By my mid-twenties I decided to let it dry naturally curly. I love the way it frames my face, shading it or balancing its roundness, or hiding it if need be. It gives me a slightly exotic look, hinting at southern Mediterranean blood. Who knows what African genes may have gotten mixed with the fairer Vendée stock when the Moors invaded the Mediterranean and Atlantic coasts of France in the eighth century.

Glasses and hair are the frames and costumes of my face, the curtains around the stage, the veils that create the illusion, the mise-en-scène. They give me something to play with, so that I can reveal or hide only as much as I choose and play as many characters as I feel like, or as suit the circumstances.

It's the head-on, flat view of my face, with hair pulled back, that I find harsher, especially with age. I prefer my three-quarters profile: more playful, more seductive, more feminine. It allows more expression, a tilt this way or that, a half smile, and the different planes of the face fall more gracefully. That is the face I prefer to present to the world. My armor, maybe. Feminine, seductive, inviting yet holding back, offering itself without giving itself away.

It has served me well, that face. It still does. I am grateful for it. I've learned to make peace with its flaws, or turn them to my advantage. I hardly see them anymore, even though age has accentuated them or created new ones. I couldn't imagine wanting to change anything about it with cosmetic surgery. I like the way it ages, even though it can look drawn and more marked when I'm tired. But it's nothing that a shot of energy and a bright smile cannot cure.

When I look at myself in the mirror, I smile. The smile corrects everything. It transcends fatigue, age, flaws. The smile is the spirit. The spirit that had flown from my mother's face when I saw her lying on the gurney. The smile makes the corners of the lips come up, forming two dimples in the cheeks. The crinkles around the eyes have resulted in crow's feet, but I like the way they look, as if my smile has created its own decorative frieze. It's that smile that has carried me through life. The smile I used to make peace between my grandparents and my mother when I was growing up, to seduce men and to be loved by them, to show my daughters that I love them, to embrace my friends, to soften the edges of my personality, to throw myself at life.

benilde little

GORGEOUS AS I THINK I AM

Every year my husband and I go on a weekend-long junket at a nice resort to celebrate the top performers in his company. At the Saturday-night dinner, a professional photographer captures each couple in a promlike stance, and the next day the pictures are displayed for us to pick up as we depart. Each year I anticipate what I'm going to look like: Maybe this time I'll finally look like myself—or, more to the point, look the way I think I do.

Never happens.

This year's picture captured a middle-aged couple. *Who the hell are they?* I'm wearing a fabulous black dress that I found in the designer section of Nordstrom, half off—still expensive, but justifiable, considering how much I wear it. Neither the dress nor my essence is captured in the

155

photograph. The question is, do I look the way I think I do, or like the photographic image? Probably the answer is both.

I've always thought of myself as attractive, and often what I see reflected in the mirror pleases me, but in pictures, different story—it's not how I think I look. I think of my face as slender, nicely sculpted, with elegant, defined cheekbones and a good chin. But it tends to look fat in pictures. Of course, personality, of which I have a lot, can't be captured on non-moving celluloid.

My dissatisfaction with this picture is nothing new. It's not about age, weight, or where we are in our marriage. It's about the reality that I am not as beautiful as I imagine myself to be in my head. I've always liked my eyes, lips, and forehead. (My brothers used to say my forehead was big, but I was never dissuaded from thinking it regal.) Those same older brothers, my torturers, also made fun of my "big schnoz." But even though my brothers taunted me, they also instilled in me a sense of invincibility. It wasn't about looks; it was more about being the youngest and the only girl, who not only took all their crap but tried, valiantly, to keep up with them. This gave me the confidence to have my own style, which is what people see when they really see me.

Growing up where and when I did—in Newark during the Black Arts movement—was a lucky break for a young black girl. I didn't lust after straight hair; I didn't get caught up in the color thing (as in, "If you white, you right; if you brown, stick around; if you black, get back"). I understood, with the help of those same brothers, that it was just colonialist nonsense, and I resisted it with all my might—all of which plays into how I see myself and go through the world. It's nearly impossible, however, to carry the weight of four hundred years' worth of being subjugated, of being seen as the mule of society, and not have some of that seep into your psyche. And yet I have weathered it better than most, thanks largely to my mother. She had impeccable, classic style and a solid sense of herself as a woman and as a black person.

Coming of age during the Blaxploitation film period in the '60s and '70s, I had many black beauty idols to look up to. Pam Grier was not only a toffee-colored beauty with a big afro and killer body, she was also tough; Diahann Carroll, the first black woman to have a TV series, *Julia*, was pretty, elegant, and competent. I had a Julia doll, friend of Barbie, complete with her white nurse's uniform and hard cap. Having idols that looked like me helped to keep me from lusting after blue eyes or blond straight hair. I understood at a very young age that each group could and should have its own standards of beauty. The image that probably had the most profound effect on me was Diana Ross as Billie Holiday in *Lady Sings the Blues*. I must have gone to see that movie at the Branford Theater in downtown Newark five times, which was a lot for a thirteen-year-old who didn't get an allowance. I was obsessed. I would dress in a gown, put a flower in my hair, and sing along with the record into a hairbrush, passing out at the end of a song while my best friend, Carolyn, laughed and applauded. I had no interest in ever being a singer (which was a good thing, since my voice sounds like a frog's with a cold), but I loved the glamour of Diana as Billie. Diana as Billie was sophisticated, strong, beautiful, and flawed. I wanted to look like her, *be* like her, minus the addiction to heroin.

My grappling with my looks began with seeing my first professionally done photograph when I was twenty-three years old. The photographer worked with me at a newspaper. He'd said he liked my look and wanted to "shoot me." I was flattered and happily agreed. He was so excited when he developed the contact sheets to show me a few days later. I too couldn't wait to see me. This was during the Brooke Shields nothing-comes-between-me-and-my-Calvins period—the jeans ads were provocative and the models pouty, and he positioned me in that vein. I imagined I'd look like the gorgeous black supermodel Beverly Johnson.

To say I was disappointed would be a serious understatement. I had such high expectations that I'd be frozen in my proper likeness in my first professionally taken photograph that I was completely unprepared for what I saw. I held the contact sheets in my hands, scanning the rows for one likeness that said *me*—but none did. Only one did me justice, an image showing half my face, giving my cheekbones that sculpted look I was so convinced was mine. That was the only one I asked to keep. The photographer gave me several, and all but one have been lost over the years.

Recently, my daughter, who is thirteen, found the remaining photograph and said, "We should frame this, Mom." "Why?" I snarled. She said, "You look really pretty." "Do you think I really look like that?" I asked her. "Kinda," she said, hunching her shoulder, letting me know the conversation was over. The truth is, the full face in that picture does look like me—even though the woman frozen in that time had no idea who she was. She wanted something big, but she wasn't sure what, or how to get it. She was trying to look serious, to be serious, but the photographer wanted sexy. There was sadness in her eyes and in her soul. It would be years before she would own it, and more before she would do something about it.

When I was a senior in college, I dated a first-year law student. I wanted to marry him, and would've done anything to make that happen. He didn't feel that way about me, though—or, as he told me, he was so focused on law school, so terrified of flunking out, that he couldn't have a "big relationship."

Years later, I'm married; he's married. He comes to a reading I'm doing at a nightclub in Washington, D.C. I read from the stage, comfortable, confident, nicely dressed in some kind of suit, hair up but still wild. He comes up to me afterward and whispers in my ear, "Can I tell you something, Bennie?" He's the only person who's ever called me that. I say sure, and he says, "You look so much better now."

I'm stunned. Did I really look so much better that he had to pull me aside to say so? I go back to my hotel room that night and stare at my image in the mirror, trying to remember, to see, the girl I'd been. I'd worn my hair in cornrows, dressed in Levi's and Brooks Brothers shirts; I'd had acne on my right cheek. My face was fuller then, but I thought I was pretty. He obviously hadn't shared that view. I wonder now: If I'd been beautiful, would he have wanted to marry me? I think about the life I would've had, marrying right out of college, and thank God for saving me from that. I was not the girl to marry right out of college, and I know that now, as surely as I sit writing this. As it turns out, "pretty but not gorgeous" has saved me, has allowed me to grow into a substantial and more interesting woman.

My daughter is tall, skinny (she still doesn't weigh a hundred pounds), graceful, and gorgeous. People look at her on the street. When we're in the mall, I'm often stopped by someone pushing some modeling offer, and I watch how packs of girls pass her and then turn around and stare. Baldwin is oblivious to most of it and, like most thirteen-year-old girls, obsesses over the tiny things: practically invisible light spots on her face, the occasional pimple. She doesn't think she's beautiful, no matter how many times strangers tell her. I'm careful to let her know that she's beautiful inside and out—that my love for her, and any other love worth having, runs much deeper than her looks. Of course, I want her to avoid the things that trip up so many women—I don't want her to waste her precious youth on silly insecurities and eating disorders.

Having a daughter who looks like Baldwin does has made it easier for me to age, to let go of a preoccupation with how I look. When we go shopping together and I try on a long, fitted T-shirt, and she tries on the same style, I say, "Oh, so *that's* how it's supposed to look." If I didn't have her, I'd probably own a lot more unflattering tight tees. I love looking at her, growing every day, and thinking, *Sweetie, it's* your *turn now.*

The other day I needed to pick up a few things at the super market, and Baldwin wanted to go with me. I agreed to let her come but told her we'd need to do it fast, before math acceleration class. She looked at me and said, in all seriousness, "You have to comb your hair first." And I said to her, "Sorry, honey, I'm going just like this." She stayed home. So here we are, mother and daughter, experiencing the same hormonal surges but at different ends: She's starting; I'm ending. She's obsessed with every single aspect of her appearance, and I am at a place where my looks—even though I may not be as gorgeous as I think I am—finally make me happy.

annaliese jakimides
LOSING FACE

It's a complicated story, this face thing. If you were to analyze all the individual components of my face—eyes, nose, lips, ears, bone structure, forehead, the overbite that is still there, even after the braces and the strap that was intended to pull the top jaw into alignment—your overall impression probably wouldn't be, *Wow, now* that's *a beautiful face.* My eyes are greenish-gold; a friend describes my nose as the most finely chiseled nose ever. I wear five earrings, often of varying lengths and designs; my hair has been crew-cut length for more than twenty years, and lately I have been dying it burgundy.

Growing up, I never saw my face as bad or homely, not beautiful or even pretty. I didn't love it. I didn't hate it. I certainly didn't want to trade it for someone else's. Bred of a jumble of Greek, French, Armenian, Irish, and possibly some Turkish genes, my face never really had an adjective in my mind.

Honestly, even as an adult I've rarely looked at my face in an attentive way. I have never defined myself by how I look, but more by how I live. I was more likely to catch sight of my reflection in the curtainless kitchen windows that separated me from the woods and pond outside my northern Maine home than in a mirror. Each morning I brushed my teeth, washed my face, maybe slapped a little powder on it, inserted the five earrings, and got going. I couldn't imagine any other way of being in the world.

And then I lost my face. Not literally, as in the world might wince at me or choose not to look in my direction if it had a choice. I lost my real face, the one I see from the inside, not the outside.

Ten years ago, my father died, my mother died, my marriage died, my children left, and a balky menopause arrived. A sudden, solitary, interminable depression stripped my face of everything I knew about it. Sorrow bled from every pore. I cried convulsively until my eyes swelled, snot running from my nose, and I choked trying to catch enough air between the sobs to breathe. I planned an exit strategy, convinced that even my children—my extraordinary children, whom I adore and who adore me—would be better off with me gone if I were like this. They didn't have to see much of the "this," since they were away at college and life, and, when needed, I could pull myself into functional mode for them, create a mask of my old self, my "real" self—I had not quite arrived at the understanding that all of it was real.

It's hard to admit even now that I was broken. Huddled in the corner on the floor of my daughter's old bedroom, frozen, curled up like a wounded dog. I cried at the checkout line at the grocery store. I could not think of the words that should come together to make a simple sentence. I slept only two hours every night. I got up, I went to work, I shopped, I washed the clothes, I wrote a few words, I forced myself to look out the window onto a world that in a past life I would have seen as brilliant, abundant, filled with possibilities, a ghost's breath of frost sweetening the glass.

A good friend tells me today that when he met me on the streets of Boston in 1967, and I smiled and said hello, he knew I was the most grounded person he would ever know. Everything I am, he says, is in my face. And that "everything" includes a joy at being in his presence, although he suspects that he is not the only one who feels that way.

He reentered my life a few years ago, after I found my face again. If he had seen me in the midst of the blackness, he would have recognized the physical face—everyone says it has changed very little over the years—but he would have been searching for the real face, the one that talked without words and loved without touch, the one that was so comfortable in the world. The one that was grounded.

During that time, it was as if yards of gauze prevented me from hearing, seeing, participating. Fuzzy, murky, watery. This face that had always been willing to open up, to take risks, to be itself anywhere, anytime, closed up on itself—no entrance into the slurry of darkness fermenting just below the surface. I couldn't let people know that I had lost myself, that the eyes I looked through registered a world of unfathomable darkness.

One day, walking out of Ken's Market on Main Street, I bumped into a woman I knew. Our children had gone to school together.

"Jackie," I said, grabbing her coat sleeve, "it's all so sad. Why is it all so sad?"

"What's so sad?" she asked.

"This life," I said. I was shocked I was saying these words, astonished at this public confession. My voice dissolved. "Just this life," I said. She stared at me as I blinked, trying unsuccessfully to fight back the swell of tears. What I saw on her face was fear masquerading as disbelief, discomfort. If I, the strong, resilient, reliable one, could crumble like this, then who might be next? Anyone might be next. She might be next.

I drove home and called the women's health center a hundred miles away. Between gulps and breaths, huge sodden heaves, I told the nurse-practitioner I couldn't stop crying. In retrospect, I can see the words were unnecessary. She gave me the name of a counselor she had used, she trusted, she could vouch for, and told me to call the minute I hung up the phone— and to call her back to tell her I had.

Oh, thank you: someone telling me what I must do. I called, and the counselor, also a hundred miles away, told me to drive down right then, that moment. The miles that mark the northernmost tip of Interstate 95 snaking down from the Canadian border are quiet and empty—like I was. Clouds hung over my old Ford Festiva, a tunnel of trees on each side. The rearview mirror was relentless and insistent. Every time I glanced up at it, I was shocked to see a woman with wet cheeks and puffy eyes, quivering lips.

After two sessions, I understood I had been like a boiling pot with the lid on, but now that it was off, there was no plunking the sucker back down on the fomenting bubbles, hot and dangerous, and no way to turn off the heat. After two sessions, I also understood how much help I needed—but I couldn't afford to keep coming back. I was at the tail end of a soon-to-be-ex-husband's health plan, and even that wouldn't cover the therapist's services, because she didn't have the right letters after her name. When I said I couldn't come again, she made me her pro bono client and kept seeing me and seeing me and seeing me. She told me she would be there for me as long as I needed her. And I needed her for a long time. She saved my life.

If I am honest, there were many who saved my life—my sons, my daughter, my friends, the clerk in the local grocery store who told me he was so happy to see my "sweet face" each time I bought an apple, some milk, cheese, no matter that I knew my face wasn't there. I hoped there was something he could see of me even if I couldn't. I, however, didn't make it easy for all the others in my life to help me. I have always known how to take care of others, fight for causes. But now I didn't even know how to take care of myself. I didn't want people to know I had lost me, couldn't find me.

One day I made a mask of my face with a friend who had recently learned how to make them by cutting up strips of material used for casts to heal broken wrists, broken arms. We cut and soaked the strips. I slathered my face with Vaseline. My friend layered the wet strips on my face, carefully working around my eyes, leaving openings for them and for my mouth. For about an hour and a half, I had to keep my face still, just breathing, looking out the holes, until my friend loosened it from my features—nose, cheeks, chin, forehead, all the skin stretched out over the bones, the malar and lachrymal; the nasal, superior, and inferior maxillary; the vomer; the turbinated and the palate bones—and placed it in my hands. I held a white mask of what I could see was a painfully sad face, my face.

Weeks turned into months. One season passed into another. Some winter nights I walked to the edge of the pond, a deep bowl of frozen ice and snow, and stood in the dark, ringed by the skeletons of birch and maple, spruce and pine, and I could think only of bones. Bone quiet, bone ash, bone dust. In spring, I caught my misshapen face in the waters, where jellylike sacks of polliwog eggs clustered along the steep banks. I balanced on the granite ledge in summer, sinking deeper and deeper. I cannot swim. In fall, I watched the fire colors of orange and crimson, yellow, float on the pond's murky surface.

Japanese avant-garde Butoh dancers assume blank faces so that they can express all the emotions of the story through the body. To use the face is like cheating. Mine could have been a perfect Butoh dancer's face—expressionless. Expressionless is not, however, what human faces are, and it is definitely not what this human face is in its natural state. One day I overheard someone saying we can choose how we greet the world, and if we greet it with even an intimation of a smile, the universe will respond in kind. I had never been a "universe" kind of person, but I was desperate. I began painfully, consciously, artificially to put on a "face" that tried to understand a reason to live. I knew that if I could just find my way back to my face, I might have a chance. And so each day, multiple times a day, I forced myself to smile just a little, to create what I thought was a face that looked like it was happy to see you. I practiced in the mirror—the mirror that I hardly ever looked in before I lost my face. Now I needed the mirror as I tried to find it again.

The suffocating gauze lifted in small, incremental pieces. I cried less. I noticed stars in the sky. Twenty-two months after the depression descended, I could recognize aspects of who I was. One day I caught a little light, a glint in my eye, as I walked by a mirror in a store. I stopped and stared at that golden-green shimmer I had known, I had lost. It's odd how the eyes can maintain their shape, their color, everything physically descriptive and recognizable, and yet lose their personality. My eyes' personality used to be glittery, funny, hopeful. Here it was again.

I passed a couple in the little park in the center of town, leaning into each other, talking. A smile began to form on my lips with no effort. I ran my fingers over its shape, feeling the way it blended into my cheeks. And then suddenly I heard a deep, staccato laugh. The couple looked in my direction and smiled. It was my laugh, coming from my mouth. It was me.

I stepped further into the world a bit tentatively, petrified that the villain of darkness could again suck my face away. No, not villain—it wasn't a villain. In truth, there have been gifts, although it took me a while to recognize them. The light is brighter, clearer now, both the incoming and the outgoing.

I think of the mask I made of my face. It sits on my living room windowsill—eventually, I painted it copper and green and gold, so it could speak "art," not "illness." It has never occurred to me that it should not speak at all. If I hold that mask up to my face now and look in the mirror, I can see the droop of the skin, the flatness and fear, the impenetrable sadness I first recognized that day in the mask as mine. It is haunting.

I have learned the larger truth of the way that every day, every experience, light and dark, weaves itself into the foundation of the next. This weaving is not a conscious action, any more than my relationship with my face is conscious. My face is shaped by every person, every emotion, every event I experience: my children, a friend's chest with its crescent scar after the mastectomy, bonfires on brittle fall nights after the last of the firewood has been cut and split and stacked, my dad in his white shirt and tie playing Legos with my son at the kitchen table, the Vietnam vet who broke my heart, the Vietnam vet who expanded it, even the two years of blinding darkness. I cannot force my face to go back to another time any more than I can give my children back, any more than I can undo love, any more than I can prevent the eruption in my pond of hundreds of thousands of polliwogs into tree frogs over the next few days.

This spring morning is wet outside the plate-glass window of the coffee shop. My face is refracted in the rain. I am visiting my thirty-two-year-old daughter in New York City, where she now lives, far from the pond and the woods in which she grew up.

"I never knew you were beautiful," she says, brushing her long, dark brown, ringleted hair away from her irrefutably beautiful face.

The coffee is steaming under her hand. She passes it over the top of the cup, warming her palm. I love the big-city energies that swirl around, all the clusters of little stories, expansive dramas, raw loves.

"But I do now," she rushes to add.

"Oh?" I ask, wondering what it is that makes this grown woman who has known me all these years suddenly and adamantly pronounce me "beautiful."

"I don't quite know how to say it, Mom. Your face lights up the room when you walk in. Oh my god, I don't believe I just said that. What a cliché."

I laugh. But I know what she means: the part of me that comes through the face, half-full, not half-empty, the me who connects with the slivers of light, the undercurrent of joy. It is a new definition of beauty for her.

marina budhos
INHERITANCE

When I was fifteen, I went for
an interview at a modeling school.
This was my brother's idea. He was a
professional musician by then, touring on the road, and he now
moved in a world of models and media and music. For some
reason, he thought it would be a good idea for his kid sister, too.
I had recently "blossomed," as they said: My braces were off,
my waist seemed to have stretched five inches, and when I went
to get my hair cut at the local salon, the hairdresser asked if he
could photograph me for their window, since my hair "showed
so well." I shrugged. The compliments gave me some pleasure
but did not sink in very much.

The modeling school was located on the second floor of a
building on Queens Boulevard. I remember my parents sitting
in chairs against the wall, looking puzzled but curious as I followed various sets of instructions. The director of the school sat

behind her desk and asked me to walk the length of the room and back to her. I did—tripping slightly on a loose flap at the bottom of my cork-wedge shoes. I remember, too, enjoying how little I cared. After all, only a few years previous, I had been a tomboy with short hair, daring the boys to climb trees. This new metamorphosis felt like a drama taking place outside of me, directed by others.

I have no idea what the director's assessment was. I do know there was some discussion about putting together a portfolio and my getting trained by the school. The place was probably no more than an amateur mill for girls with hopelessly impossible ambitions—no different from the dance or music schools that adorned the same avenue, promising another kind of life on the magical island of Manhattan, just a few miles away. My heart wasn't in it, though, and I think my parents were relieved not to spend the money.

But that idea—that I was supposed to "do" something with my looks—never really disappeared. In fact, the notion had been planted so early on that it was hard to disregard. It was there before I was born, in fact, when my mother—a spirited, rebellious daughter of Orthodox Jews—defied her family by marrying the man she called her "handsome movie star"—an Indian graduate student from the Caribbean. For my mother, her children's exotic looks became a way to stand out, to be different, and to chart a more exciting, unusual path for our family.

We moved to Parkway Village, a garden-apartment community in Queens, when I was four years old. Originally built for UN families, Parkway became a magnet for mixed families during the '60s and '70s, a refuge of racial integration. Parkway kids were part black, part Japanese, part Scandinavian, mixed-race exotics, long before chic Benetton ads or superstars like Tiger Woods or Barack Obama. I wasn't even the only half-Indian, half-Jewish girl in Parkway: There was Maya Bhatt, who wore her hair straight down to her butt and looked like my twin sister. And there was Bimla Dindial, exactly the kind of girl my brother hoped I would become: She knew how to carry herself, both aloof and warm, with a casual sense of fashion. I remember she was the first teenager to wear a camel-hair coat, cinched at the waist. Her friends were often older, foreign; Bimla seemed destined for fashion and money. She and my brother dated for a brief while, and she seemed the perfect accessory for his maroon convertible Triumph.

At home, our cultural mixture was supposed to be a passport to a grander, more special, more exciting life. My mother would page through advertisements in magazines and point out which models resembled my brother and me; she'd tell me that when I grew up I'd be either Marlo Thomas or Cher—both mysterious ethnic beauties on TV. When I became a teenager, my mother loved to exclaim: "You have breasts, not like me!" When we went shopping on Jamaica Avenue, a mostly black and West Indian neighborhood, she'd nudge and whisper, "Did you see how they looked at you!" My mother experienced a strange, vicarious thrill through the looks of her children. It was her passport to other racial worlds, to glamour. And it was my inheritance, a gift I felt I was supposed to act upon.

Certainly, there was a whiff of compensation, of insecurity, in my mother's comments. I suppose my mother thought she was doing something good for our self-worth. Being a Parkway kid meant being part of a sweet, idealistic moment. We grew up remarkably insulated from prejudice. At a time when the country was much more racially divided, and mixed-race children might have felt confused or ugly or different, we felt quite the opposite. We felt superior. Dark was different, better, special. To be black or brown was cool. White or conventional prettiness, like on TV, was boring, unattractive, conformist. I didn't even know we were supposed to feel badly about ourselves.

And so we Parkway kids were special, foreign without being too foreign. We were the kids who could cross over and make it in the gleaming world of America for our differentness—indeed, it was our difference that made us special. Parkway was a magnet for kids from other neighborhoods; they would cluster on our village green at night, smoking pot and envying us our cosmopolitan environs. We were the center; we were beautiful, crossing back and forth between black, brown, and white worlds.

It was also the times—most of us in Parkway were keenly aware of fashion and rebellious coolness. Our family spent summers in England, where my brother would go to King's Road and spend all his money on suede Beatle boots. One summer he lived in Liverpool with a Parkway friend who looked like Jimi Hendrix; I remember my brother showing up at my aunt and uncle's door in a dramatic velvet cape that swirled to his knees. I wore his hand-me-downs: shaggy deerskin jackets, faded work shirts. At school I copied the black girls, with their wedge shoes and bell-bottoms, and learned how to dance the hustle.

My brother became the anti-intellectual rebel; girls fell for his dark looks, his aloofness, his intensity. He also had another gift—music, which became his passport to making it in

America. Much to my immigrant father's dismay, he dropped out of college and began touring as a musician. The phone would ring all the time with calls from other musicians. He would call people "cat" and talk about "sessions." He was fulfilling my mother's fantasies—that we could stand out and count in the world, through the arts, our looks, and charisma.

But what was all that to me?

I was the free-spirited kid sister who half-dreamed about entertainment. In the privacy of my small bedroom, I wrote stories and screenplays. I memorized TV shows and revered *The Brady Bunch*. All of this cohered into a vague idea of going to Hollywood, so I wrote to the head of CBS and asked him how I could become a TV actress. For me, these drama fantasies were also a way of leaving my mixed-up, mixed-race, half-foreign world; of crossing over, shooting past Queens Boulevard, over the 59th Street Bridge, to the silvery Oz of Manhattan and "making it," like all those figures my mother seemed to admire.

And I even showed some real determination: When the sixth-grade graduation play was *Oliver*, I organized a rebellion, demanding that girls get to play parts in Fagin's gang. I secretly plotted to take over the role of the Artful Dodger, perfecting my cockney accent and actually succeeding, to thunderous applause.

Despite that burning moment of stardom, though, I was mostly shy and bookish, preferring to disappear into novels and art, thinking and writing. Indeed, my moment of seizing the limelight was driven by a mission of fairness and ideas— that girls be given plum roles too. And it was in school that I felt most alive and seen. But with my brother, the dark comet blazing a different path, my gifts seemed almost a liability, an embarrassing conformism.

When it came time for junior high, those of us in the academically gifted classes were given a choice of skipping eighth grade. That's what I wanted to do, as I'd been with the same group of kids—mostly smart, Jewish kids destined for the magnet high schools and competitive colleges—since kindergarten. But my parents sent my brother upstairs to talk me out of the accelerated program.

"That's for nerds," my brother told me. "My friends, we laugh at them." What he meant was: Don't hang around with those short, nerdy, Jewish science-and-math types headed to Stuyvesant. I was supposed to be attractive and popular, to have a mysterious power over people, as he did. I think he was actually worried that I was falling behind on the social scale—which I was—and that I would not be cool, like he was.

While my parents probably didn't know exactly what my brother would say to me, his warnings accorded with their own sentiment that their "little girl" shouldn't go so far away from them, taking a long subway ride to go to school with the pushy kids of overbearing parents.

Beneath lay another tension: my being good at academics threatened my mother. For most of my childhood, she had struggled to finish her undergraduate degree, then her master's, and she was now hoping to pursue a PhD. She too was a voracious reader, yet it was never something we could share. Like everything she did, she worked hard and obsessively, even possessively—literature and academics were hers, and we never developed a language for sharing ideas and thoughts, perhaps because she feared I would eclipse her at the very moment she was seeking her own expression. When it came to intellectual matters, she was to command the stage, and I was supposed to fill in at the edges. I knew, in some deep part of myself, that my family wanted compliance from me—that I was to stay within their orbit, their idea of who I was. Being academically aggressive didn't fit with the cool, above-it-all, attractive image of my family. We were supposed to shoot past ordinary aspirations, to exotic fame.

So I followed my family's wishes. I didn't skip a grade, nor did I try out for the magnet high schools. I dropped my old friends and drifted. For a brief while, I affected a rebellious persona, a shadow image of my brother's. I joined the theater program in high school, cut classes, and hung around Greenwich Village, watching double matinees of foreign films. I wore vintage clothes—jackets from the '40s with padded shoulders and rhinestone buttons, army–navy berets and sailor pants— and kept up a secret intellectual life, poring over Jean Genet on the subway and trying to understand what *Waiting for Godot* was really about.

When it came time to decide on college, I was confused. Still lingering in my mind were inchoate ambitions around theater and "being someone." And yet I kept wishing I could just go to a solid college for a few years. I wanted to be normal, like my other friends, who were packing up for dorm life and picking out the usual fare of freshman classes. They seemed younger than I, unburdened.

I chose the NYU drama program, which pleased everyone. My parents bought my brother and me a cramped apartment in

Chelsea—he worked on his music career, and I went to classes downtown. It was all a movie set: I saw myself jogging around Washington Square Park, talking to interesting boys in cafés. I was aware, somehow, that I was supposed to be fulfilling a fantasy of a young woman let loose in New York City—perhaps finally catching up to my brother's standards of coolness. So I would experiment to see if I could attract young men. And I did—at the library, in cafés—and then I would obligingly meet them for chaste, nervous dates. My experimentation with using my looks to get attention was far more interesting than the encounters themselves, which often filled me with a heavy dread.

I got a job at an art gallery, where everyone seemed sophisticated and sexually knowing. One woman gave us tips on how to use one's eyes to attract men; another revealed that she sewed expensive labels into cheap coats and then casually draped them across a chair. The curator, a quirky red-haired woman, owned the most spectacular collection of Tony Lama cowboy boots. So I saved up my money and spent $400 on a pair of exquisite maroon cowboy boots—an unfathomable sum at the time. I loved wearing them as part of my tough, New York City fashion-girl image; I polished them weekly with a chamois cloth and colored mousse.

But within six weeks at NYU, I also knew I was not meant for the theater. My New York City life—orchestrated with my parents' approval—was starting to feel like a skiddy surface I would eventually crash on. I hated everything about the program. I hated that we didn't talk about plays in depth; I was bored by my acting classes. Yes, I wanted to be someone; I loved clothes and urban fashion and glamour, but I had no drive to make use of my adult body onstage. Mostly I floated through the program, feeling naive and foolish. There was a sweet sincerity to my Parkway upbringing, an innocence, and I was completely unprepared for the kind of hard-edged striving that surrounded me. I felt as if I were eight years old, still peering at *The Brady Bunch*, wishing I could be on that screen.

One night, I was hanging out at the apartment of a fellow student, smoking pot and eating from tiny boxes of food brought from Balducci's, where she worked. This girl mesmerized and repelled me: She had jet-black short hair and dressed in severe clothes; her apartment was a studio she shared with a roommate, and it was fashionably white all over—white walls, white chairs, huge white bed. We were comparing notes on our teachers and classes when she suddenly announced, "I'm going to sleep with our voice teacher."

When she saw my look of shock, she assured me, "That's how you get ahead in this business."

That night I walked home, shaken and stoned, past Washington Square Park and 8th Street, where I loved to cruise for fashionable shoes, and said to myself: *I am getting out, as soon as I can.*

Theater, I realized, was not just a gift, something natural. It was hard, conscious work. Cynical work, in this girl's case. Those around me in the drama program burned with a real desire to thrust themselves forward, in public. I burned too, but my desire had nothing to do with moving myself across a stage or in front of a camera. The little girl who enjoyed acting out TV shows in the privacy of her bedroom actually didn't have the hunger to do so in public. This wasn't the same as prancing on the sixth-grade stage as the Artful Dodger. This entailed an adult knowingness, using beauty and sexuality, that made me uncomfortable.

Not long after, I was having lunch with another friend, Julia. She was a brilliant private-school Manhattan kid who already knew she wanted to be an avant-garde director—my first intellectual friend. When I told her I wanted to transfer from NYU, she said, "Why don't you try Cornell or Brown? That's where a lot of my friends want to go."

Little did Julia know, she changed my life. She helped me start to turn away from that vague promise of my skin, to what was inside.

So I wrote the names down. At the time, I did not even know what an Ivy League college was. I just knew I had to get away. I wrote a long, heartfelt admissions essay about how I'd messed around in high school, but now I wanted to be a writer.

When I read the essay out loud to my mother, she said, "You don't have to be so negative."

But I did feel negative. I felt that I had squandered the other inheritance—that of the gift of creating, writing, and thinking.

In the end, I chose Cornell and decided to take a semester off, working as a waitress in a café in Chelsea. One day, a young man gave me a card. He was a photographer, and he was interested in photographing me with some turquoise jewelry for his portfolio.

I was curious. It was as if I was following through on that modeling-school interview years ago, opening a door on that other life. After checking out his references a few days later, at his studio a block away, I tried out my modeling fantasy.

Beneath shiny white umbrellas, I wrapped myself tightly in a towel, showing my bare arms and neck, letting down my hair. The turquoise-and-silver jewelry was too chunky for me. But he took other shots. And as the camera clicked away, I became aware that I could pose more—throw back my hair, go toward the camera. I could make use of that inheritance, a way of seducing, drawing upon what I had observed in those other, more glamorous Parkway girls.

And yet I couldn't. Some part of me rebelled, knew this was part of the pliancy that had always been expected of me as the dark-eyed, good daughter. Ironically, that which my mother gave me—the gift of intellect—she did not want to see. And so, in a way, I had allowed myself to be stilled, to be something that was looked at. And to go toward this life would muffle something else—an inner, stubborn, fighting voice that was dying to come out; to talk, express, and analyze.

Years before, when I walked across the office of the modeling school, it was a lark, trying out a story born from other people's desires. But it was not my story. And I finally knew that. Models, I realized, speak with their bodies. Those with a glamorous allure exert a kind of quiet control; they are rarely garrulous, knowing how to leave a tantalizing space in between. But the truth was, I didn't like eyes on me, and I didn't like using my body as an instrument of expression. I preferred being the observer, the recorder and thinker. What my mother saw as a passport to the world had become a hindrance to me.

So that day, under the warm glare of bulbs, I felt the rush of words. I began to talk to the photographer about the mechanics of lighting, as if willing myself to the other side of the camera. I knew there was no frisson, no erotics of looking, for I consciously pressed it down.

I knew, too, that if I ever seriously pursued modeling or acting, I would be forced to put myself under harsh scrutiny, enduring a whole set of gradations and judgments: the nose that was too long, with its bump on the bridge; the slightly pursed mouth that would never be lush enough; the overbite, for my teeth had shifted from orthodontia. I was thin but not model thin. I didn't have that leggy walk. My hands and feet were strong, not delicate and bony; my shoulders were too broad. It was easier to float in a sweet bubble of self-worth, the childish glamour fantasy that Parkway had given me, than to get serious about such a career. Fashion, modeling, theater were just too much work for something I did not want badly enough. Besides, the era I had been born into—when Parkway kids were exotics— was passing. More and more, I'd see other young people who looked like me, and it was with some relief that I could blend and not feel the pressure to be different.

About a week later, the photographer came into the café with his contact sheets, excited. He had shared them with a friend in advertising, who wanted me to pose for an Air Jamaica ad. I knew what he meant: a wet-T-shirt ad. I smiled, felt flattered and repelled, and took the number. But I never called.

Shortly before I left for Cornell, I sold my prized maroon cowboy boots and bought a pair of utterly ugly L.L.Bean boots, which I never wore. It didn't matter. At the time, I was willing myself into a preppy college identity. I wanted to think, to go inside and forget my skin.

That evening, as I watched my buyer walk off with my

gorgeous boots, marked the end of my toying with being a model or an actress. There was something more I wanted, an inner drive that had yet to find its form on the outside. Of course, I had new fantasies: I would be a brilliant director, staging provocative Marxist and feminist plays, my bearded graduate-student boyfriend by my side. Most of all, I was leaving what I knew: the inheritance of my family, of Parkway, setting out in a cold January to figure out who I could be in the world.

pamela redmond satran
OPEN MOUTH

"Close your mouth," the photographer or the make-up artist or the dental hygienist says.

I try, even though I know that it doesn't really close. And it doesn't: Even closing my mouth, as a test to write these sentences, drawing in air, is an unfamiliar experience, my lower lip catching on my upper teeth, like a foot tripping on a stair that's too tall. I force my upper lip down, the muscles weak, ineffective. I press my lips together, briefly, incompletely.

And then my mouth pops open again, and I'm drawing air in, despite lifelong instructions not to be a mouth breather: A hole that big can't just sit there doing nothing. At least I'm comfortable, if noncompliant.

"It doesn't really close," I explain. "I have a short upper lip."

"You have witch's teeth," a small child said to me once, gazing at my mouth in awe and horror.

I must have looked stricken, because the child (who was undoubtedly a child with whom I had some kind of warm relationship, though I've repressed the child's identity along with, no doubt, my wish to smother her) recovered and said, "They're nice witch's teeth, though."

They're not really witch's teeth, I hope, *because witch's teeth are green,* I think, *and pointy.* They're not quite Bugs Bunny teeth either: They stick out farther than that. They're just long and prominent and tending toward yellow, though I had them bleached a few years ago in what even my twelve-year-old son called my most transformational beauty and/or fashion move of all time.

It isn't just my teeth that are the problem, anyway, or my short upper lip: It's my whole mouth. I have a big smile, a huge smile, a smile that's one of my best qualities, except for the vast acreage of gum that it exposes. My gums, thanks to the dentist with whom I've become so familiar that he kisses me hello and calls me "girlfriend," are at least in better shape than they used to be. For years, despite the fact that it was exposed at all times to all viewers, my mouth was a place I never wanted to look.

"Do you brush your teeth?" my brother once asked me.

I clapped my hand over my mouth and cried, "Of course I brush my teeth!"

But I didn't really brush them closely or carefully, not wanting to get too close to the mirror, feeling uneasy about probing my gumline, and completely unwilling to do anything like floss. I was as freaked out about the idea of peering too deeply into my own mouth as some women are about inspecting their vaginas.

Why? I can guess. I suffered through braces, at a tender age, with a cut-rate orthodontist who was more interested in chasing his pink-haired nurse around the chair than in taking care of my teeth. He pulled teeth with no anesthetic; I remember the pain of Novocain needles and whirring drills. My mother was terrified of the dentist too, opting to have all her teeth replaced with false ones when she was in her fifties.

And anatomy is destiny, so even before I was traumatized by the dental profession and by my own parent, the configuration of my mouth prompted a full range of fears and insecurities. Tripping and falling—a fairly regular occurrence, since I had pigeon toes as well as an overbite—often involved chomping down on my lip and banging my front teeth. In fact, for a long time, I had a recurring nightmare of falling off a curb and knocking my teeth clear out of my head.

As a young adolescent, I was morbidly self-conscious about my mouth: Did I have gunk on my teeth? Food between them? While the dread braces at least short-circuited any Bugs Bunny jokes, I still compulsively shielded my mouth with my hand, not wanting to give anyone else a look. I didn't want to look either; I focused on my eyes or my hair or my skin in the mirror—anywhere but my mouth. The less I saw, the better I was able to fool myself into believing that everything was fine.

It went deeper than that, of course. It wasn't only my faulty mouth and teeth I wanted to cover up and ignore; it was all the shaky underpinnings of my life: my mother's rheumatoid arthritis, which rendered her bedridden. My boyfriend's possessiveness and rage. The fact that I was desperate to leave home but had no money and no idea how to get away.

So I closed my eyes and tuned out danger, ignored pain, and leapt, hoping that everything would be all right. That's how I left my family, and made my way through college, and married and then divorced my jealous boyfriend, and moved to New York and launched a career and had children and weathered the deaths of my parents and brother.

And then my mouth started to fall apart. Fillings popped out, gums caved in, roots withered, teeth cracked in half. Worse, I was so scared of the dentist—and went through so many awful dentists—that I had to take sedatives not only before but *after* each visit (that is, when I could work up the nerve to visit at all). The time we spent living in California, where nitrous flowed freely in every dentist's office, helped shore me up, but our years in England, where a dentist once dropped a gold crown down my throat and then performed the Heimlich maneuver to bring it back up, were a serious setback.

But there came a time, with maturity and life experience, I suppose, when I finally got brave enough to look into my mouth. What I saw wasn't pretty. My gums were inflamed, my teeth were falling apart, and I had no choice but to take serious charge. Hands trembling and heart pounding, I asked everyone I knew for dentist recommendations, and even some people I didn't know, including *New York Times* science writer Natalie Angier, whom I emailed for the name of her dentist after she wrote about being dentist-phobic.

One of these recommendations led me to Dr. Z, a.k.a. The Most Expensive Dentist in the World. When I confessed my dental fears to Dr. Z, he brushed them aside, saying, "I'll cure you of that."

And he did, not primarily because he was a fabulous dentist—though he was—but because he was the perfect combination of kind and confident. Here's what you need, he'd tell me, here's how I'm going to do it, and here's some extra nitrous to help you cope. After a few months, the only thing that really made me nervous was opening Dr. Z's bill.

In two years of visiting Dr. Z, I spent $40,000 on my mouth. I had a bone graft, three extractions, four implants, seven root canals, and more crowns than I can count. Dr. Z moved to a plush new office on floor thirty-something of a building on Manhattan's East Side. I got everything fixed that ever needed to be fixed *and* became comfortable with gazing at my molars in the mirror. I even learned to floss. Learned to *like* flossing.

Getting a grip on my mouth inspired me to take charge of other, less frightening aspects of my life—the rest of my body, for instance. I lost thirty-five pounds after I got my teeth fixed. After suffering through a bone graft, after all, how hard could it be to eat less chocolate and take more walks? What I was writing got deeper too, once I'd become more willing to explore the source of my pain and expose it to the light.

My marriage changed along with my teeth. I found myself wanting to examine problems I'd swallowed for years, feeling at last as if it was preferable to work things through, however torturous the process, than to pretend they didn't exist. My adventures in extreme dentistry made me brave enough to go into therapy (the therapist's probe was far less sharp than the dentist's) and out again, virtual smile rehabilitated. While all of my deeper issues may not be resolved, at least I've examined them from all sides and know what kind of work they could still use.

The thousands I spent on dentistry didn't give me a cosmetically perfect mouth. That may be the American ideal, but it's never been mine. Strong is more important than straight, healthy to the core is preferable to a flawless veneer.

The only thing Dr. Z couldn't fix was my short upper lip, and therefore my terminally open mouth. But at least these days, the view that's always on display is more attractive. My outsize teeth might still look scary to a five-year-old, but they're solidly rooted in my gums, and my gums hardly ever bleed.

Now, when I look in the mirror and see my permanently open mouth, I'm reminded not of my vulnerabilities, but that I've never faced a problem I couldn't handle. And though it might seem impossible, my smile gets even bigger.

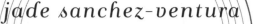

jade sanchez-ventura

IN SPITE OF MY SKIN

In public, I watch them watch-
ing me. I walk alone through the
city where I live, down streets familiar
to me from childhood, and I feel a gaze follow that does not
falter but is always watching, desiring the face I walk behind.
Here is a face, but I had no say in it. It is a thing that was done
to me. It is the thing to which I am confined.

Men watch, liking this face that was assembled for me.
This pretty face given me, and I am walking and they watch
me—here comes this pretty young thing.

"What are you?" they ask.

To answer, I open my mouth, inhale, but "I" is not my first
word. To answer I speak of other people.

"My mother is. . . . My father is. . . . "

"That's a good combination," they say, looking me up
and down again. Appraising, then approving. Or, "That's

some combination," and they are surprised and they are looking me up and down.

When they ask, they ask because they sense something—some brown man somewhere.

When they ask, it's because they want to look at me longer, and then my answer is convenient, their way in: "That's a good combination."

I *am* grateful for the accident of beauty. But I'm sure I take it for granted. I can tell, because I resent it. Not it, not the beauty itself, but how it counts for something, as if it were a quality, as if it tells something essential about me. But how can it? All it is is an accident. All it is are those mysteries of long-dead kin, collected in my body and made into something new. A face. I am not responsible. I did nothing.

The same words in ever-changing combinations: "My mother's family is from Norway and Sweden. . . . My father was born in Mexico City. . . . My mother is white . . . from the Midwest . . . divorced. . . . His parents are from Spain . . . single mother . . . I grew up in Brooklyn . . . mixed . . . he's not white."

My skin is a problem.

My parents married in a Texas courthouse when I was two years old. We were driving from Mexico to Illinois, and they were trying to appease my mother's relatives, who would not accept an illegitimate child. The divorce came two years later, when I was four. My mother and I then moved from Illinois to New York, and my father left, to Spain I think. He visited once every year, always in the spring. The visits were never planned;

he'd just appear. He was difficult to reach, nomadic; he lived in Pennsylvania, California, Mexico. He skipped one year. I remember it because of the sentence, bragging almost, in the schoolyard: "I haven't see my father in two years."

His visits lasted a few weeks, and every day we played baseball. And even though we both knew I was a shortstop, he trained me to play every position in the field, it being important to him that I know the philosophy of each one. In the late afternoons, we'd sit and watch the teenage boys compete in neighborhood-league games. He'd narrate the plays, explaining strategy so that when the time came, I'd be ready to play on a team.

"When you're in high school, your boyfriends will come and watch you play ball. Promise me, eh?"

And I promised.

I was a pretty child, and I'm sure it made him happy.

"They say I look like my father's mother," I say sometimes, when I am explaining. And I speak of him like this, not lying but telling parts of true things, which is more dangerous than lying. I can almost be convinced of the things I say, these implications of a family that does not exist. Because there is no "they," because that grandmother was dead before I was born, because now, at age twenty-six, I haven't seen my father in thirteen years.

My secret: I court the sun sometimes, looking to it to darken my face, lift off a layer of whiteness and reveal my father below.

When I was eleven, I got some local teenage girls angry at me. My mother and I lived in an apartment building on a busy avenue in Brooklyn. The neighborhood was changing around us, and we were part of the change—white artists and families moving in gradually, searching for cheap rent, liking the park up the hill and avoiding certain blocks after dark. We knew our neighbors, ate on credit at the Chinese restaurant on the corner, chatted with the couple who ran the butcher shop.

When the girls came looking for me the third time, my mother called the cops. The cops told my mother to take a Valium and get a gun. She bummed a Camel Filter off them, her first in a year, and sat smoking in the kitchen after they left. Thinking only of fleeing and protecting me, she moved us out of our apartment. The whole process took about a week.

It was spring, my father's season, and the week after we moved, he appeared for his annual visit and discovered us gone. My mother had left a letter for him with a friend, explaining the move, saying that he could reach us at my grandmother's. She wrote the phone number in the letter.

This was the moment it all changed. When he called my grandmother's house, he was furious, convinced my mother was trying to cut him out and take me from him. I've never understood this, because she'd left the letter to tell him where we were.

Things didn't get better. Every time we talked, he was yelling. He began to demand things he had never wanted before, like regular visitation and weekends away together. He told us he wouldn't leave the country until he got what he wanted. This might have been welcomed if he weren't so frightening. I didn't want to be alone with him.

His was a self-fulfilling prophecy. His anger was overwhelming, and in trying to avoid it, we began to hide from him.

He wrote constantly, called often. I had no defenses against the onslaught of letters and calls. I felt myself dissolving, and after two years, I stopped speaking to him by phone. My mother saved the letters so I could read them later.

The last time I saw my father was my first day of high school. I was fourteen.

The day had passed like a parade. We freshman girls walked through the hallways, the glances of the older boys falling like confetti among us—caught in our hair, on our lips, on the cuffs of our new jeans.

My smile was broad; my teeth sparkled beneath the fluorescent lights. I felt their eyes on me. I felt myself radiating heat, an aura of sex. I wanted them to watch me, and they knew. We recognized in each other a mutual wanting. This first day was the first time I knew boys to really watch me.

After school, I stood on the corner with three of my girlfriends, smoking maybe my tenth cigarette ever, when I looked up and into the angry eyes of my father. I hadn't seen him in months. He stood across the street, and his brown eyes were humming, furious. He always looked like a fallen king when he was angry—proud and wronged. We stared at each other, and then I turned and ran away, sprinting down the block toward my school.

I know why I ran. Seeing him, I felt only his fury and my fear. My friend Roz remembers it like a movie, like the scene when the bad guy appears, and then a van passes and he's gone. I still ask her to describe it sometimes, always relieved that she was scared too. Because though I know why I ran, I don't know where that fear came from, or rather, my reasons for it have never been good enough. There's never been one thing I could point to—a violent act, anything—to justify that moment of my turning my back and running from him.

That first day of high school, the silence began, and the count: Two weeks since. Six months. Three years. No letters, no phone calls, no sign of him. My mother and I knew nothing of where he was.

I began to watch for him everywhere, always with half an eye out. When I caught glimpses of men who looked like him—dark men with curling hair, a round belly, and my same brown eyes—I wanted it to be him as much as I was afraid it was.

As I moved further into teenagehood, I began to see it was possible for my father to disappear altogether. My body barely holding on to him, my skin too white to give proof of him, the only way to make him exist would be to speak of him, but what would I say? *He's gone, I don't know where he is, I don't think he's coming back. I was frightened of him, I ran away. He's from Mexico. In Mexico, maybe.*

I feel a gaze follow me, and I imagine an audience behind it, ever watching and judging. I say out loud that I hate this gaze, but what I don't say is what I need from it, how much I look to it for an answer. I want to know its ruling. I want it to tell me what it sees.

My whiteness feels like the second betrayal.

Seven years later, when I was a junior in college, I decided to look for my father. The silence of the past seven years had become a sadness like fog, punctured by bouts of paralyzing anxiety. I thought if I found him, I might find my way out of it.

I found him on the Internet. I emailed him, and he wrote back. In our letters, we spoke of love, of our joy at being in contact again. He thanked me for finding him. He had given up on me, he said. I broke his heart, he said, when I ran from him. He'd returned to Mexico and assumed he would never see me again.

I began dreaming of traveling to Mexico, picturing again and again the moment in the airport when he would meet me, admire my long hair, hug me. In this fantasy, I tried to blur out the figure of the friend I'd have to bring with me, but the shape of that person remained, the intrusion of my fears into even my imagined world. I couldn't help knowing I'd always be too scared to see him alone.

Our email correspondence was punctuated by a few phone calls. The first was wonderful, brief. Nobody said my name the way he did. But with each additional call, I became more uneasy. I didn't like how I felt with his voice in my ear. I became like a young child, weak, his voice just exactly the same as I remembered it, and I felt I would do anything to believe in his love.

For two years, we exchanged letters, and it was good. He gave me the words I wanted. But then his letters changed. His words became vicious. I don't know why. He told me it was time to give up on this Spanish father–American daughter thing. He called me unfeeling, told me I didn't really love him. I felt the dissolution begin, the sadness edge back in—but this time, I saw that he had never been around. That once a year had never been enough. That he'd chosen, and he hadn't chosen me. He told me, as he had many times in many emails, that he forgave me for running that day. I saw, too, that being perpetually forgiven means that I will always be blamed.

He has been the gatekeeper to a culture I seek, and he has not let me pass. My *gringa* mother has given me what she could of Mexico. She tells me of the avocado tree in the garden, of my friend, a girl named Mariposa. *Mariposa* means "butterfly." I know because my mother told me. She tells me of the markets where she walked, tall and blond. She carried me on her hip and from her hand dangled the small blue bucket to carry home the cornmeal. She tells me how my first words were in Spanish, and how I continued to ask for *agua* for years.

And she is the one who tells me about his family: his mother, whose roots were in northern Africa. This is the connection that must be the cause of his dark skin—not black, but brown— the long-ago people, consumed by a long-ago empire, whose genes reassert themselves in the children of the children of the empire. The surprise of the *negrito* or *negrita*, the little dark ones born to lighter-skinned parents. And so my father is one and I am not.

When I was young, he'd tell me to be proud of all the cultures I held in my body. But now, in turning away from me, he's telling me I don't belong.

If I were darker, he would have to let me in. He'd have to. Or maybe, too, I wouldn't need his permission. His approval. Him. Because the skin would be something no one could deny.

In my last letters, I asked him, over and over, to explain: "Why are you so mean to me? Why are you angry at me?" He told me he wasn't, that he was simply telling me the truth, that I was not Mexican like he and my cousins; that I was white, and only white, American, nothing like him—and that sometimes the truth is painful. "I love you," he wrote. "I always will." And then, in the same email, he told me that he will delete all my emails before he reads them. He will not see me.

Like a scream. What am I? What can I be if I have nothing of the people who gave me half my body? The blood is not enough. I need more if I'm going to understand this body that holds me, my witnessed self, for which I have no explanation that I want to share.

Until now, my father has suffused my body with his anger, his temper, his denial. I have carried the story of my father in my skin, behind my face. He has loaded this body with meanings that I do not understand.

When I first wrote him as an adult, I thought it was a beginning. I thought he would tell me his stories, that he would explain his family to me, his life, where he came from. I looked to him to decipher my body for me.

I now know he never will. I now know that the man I was hoping to find may not ever have existed. Strangely, losing my idea of him is as painful as the current silence between us. Before, even in my fear, I believed there was a time that had been good, a time to which we could return. If I had run from it, then maybe I could run back to it. I know now that the past holds no more than the present, the one in which I'm learning to use the word "estranged."

"I am estranged from my father."

"We are estranged."

"We have an estrangement."

He is a stranger.

It can be lonely.

I need to learn my body without him. It's time for me to go to Mexico alone; to accept that I'll find out his mother's name only from a bureaucrat's impersonal records; to gradually, I hope, assemble a new way of knowing my body.

For now, I hate that I still search my face for signs of him. He has dismissed me, and it is within his power to do so. His body is in me, but mine is not in his. And so if I can't have him, then I want to be free of him. I want him to not matter, to be powerless, to be meaningless. Maybe nothing would be better than these traces and hints that require me to explain and talk about him and keep him ever present, a reminder of what I don't have, maybe never did. I want to not need him. I want him to be a fleck of dust, and I flick him, and he is gone, and then I can be alone.

susan davis

SUDDENLY

*When I was just shy of eigh-
teen,* my surgeon father lost his
patience with my snoring and hauled
me off to an ear/nose/throat doctor. A completely benign tumor
was growing in the cartilage between my nostrils, and would
eventually plug my nose. "Okay," we all agreed, "let's have it removed." The nice doctor also suggested, "Why don't you think
about having the outside fixed as well?" *Fixed? Isn't removing
the tumor the fix?* He sent us to see a plastic surgeon.

The disproportionate size of my nose—its sloping, hooked
dominance over the rest of my face—was not news to me. The
objective ugliness of the thing and my consequential ugliness had been an unabashed topic of conversation and tool for
mockery since puberty. (In the sixth grade, nearly everyone
signed my yearbook, "To Schnoz. . . . ") But until the discovery
of the tumor, my nose had always *worked*. And because it was,

beyond a doubt, a rather extreme but sincere replica of my father's nose, I considered it to be among the unfortunate spoils of my inheritance. As my small-nosed sister liked to quip, "It comes with the brains."

So began a series of visits with a soft-spoken plastic surgeon, bearing an impossibly long last name, who specialized in cleft palates. (I was consistently the oldest patient in his waiting room—imagine sitting somewhere lit only by diffused sunlight and the neon glow from a fish tank, with scattered toys and ten to fifteen worried mothers bouncing oblivious babies on their knees, each child with a mouth that looked like it had been split with a meat cleaver.) The plastic surgeon was a friend of my father's and had, at least twice, sewn my brother's fingers back on after investigations into lawn mowers and the garbage disposal. I trusted him because he respected me. He sketched my face several times, took pictures, and asked me questions. He concluded that my nose, besides being too big, was too "masculine." He would lessen everything and round the sharp places, softening. He would leave the imperfections. Since my nostrils were naturally two different sizes, they would stay that way. He promised not to craft my nose into an assembly-line version of "cute." He liked to talk about a nose's "personality." He was wonderful. I was a teenager who had lived by my wit and style and was fiercely attached to my individuality. I didn't want a "nose-job nose." I let him operate. Years later, when he died in a small-plane crash, I had trouble explaining why I cried and cried.

Agreeing to surgery was neither an easy nor a simple decision. I had lived a long time as a religious and cultural stereotype. I'm Jewish. I had a *big* Jewish nose. My brother has this same nose and suffered for it as well, although differently. He was rarely insulted as ugly, but was subjected to the usual idiotic comments, like "So, do you only have to take one breath a day?" It was like a boy who's unusually tall or has ridiculously big feet: It was an oddity, but it didn't define him.

It defined me. Yet he and I are each an interesting study in compensatory behavior. Neither of us grew up pretty, but he grew up athletic and sociable, and I grew up smart and funny. I'd like to say that I cultivated my intelligence because it was rewarding, but actually, I felt I had no other choice. Reading was something I could do alone, without mirrors or disapproving eyes. My parents were loving, admiring people, but they made no mention of my attractiveness. (To their credit, they made no mention of my unattractiveness, either.)

Once, while shopping with my mother, I heard her behind me greet someone from her past. When the woman said, "Is this your daughter?" my mother spun me around to say hello. The woman looked at me, then at my conventionally pretty mother, then back at me, then at my mother again, and said, "Oh, I'm so sorry," before walking away. To be sure, I was not malformed, but it's important to know that my mother was (and is) quite pretty, with clear blue eyes and high cheekbones, creamy skin, and a lovely, proud, regal nose. In fact, my mother has exactly the nose many nose-job patients want. So it often surprised people how dramatically I did *not* resemble my pretty mother. That was the implied tragedy, that I looked exactly like a big-nosed Jewish man. I was not a broken-spirited girl; I had a strong sense of myself as being smart and full of good humor—

compensation for my nose. Yet I was also often melancholy and lonely—feelings I thought were punishment for my nose.

Thanks to the tumor, insurance paid for the surgery, so we didn't have money issues. We did have political issues. My mother was (and is) a committed, active feminist, and she filled our house with like-minded women, books, and conversation. They were what are now called "choice feminists"— Gloria Steinem types who believed that what women did and called "empowering" was, in fact, empowering. I knew quite a bit about the patriarchy at seventeen, and I was even voted "most liberated woman" in my high school graduating class. I knew that elective plastic surgery topped the list of capitulations to patriarchal notions of beauty. And besides, it was mutilation.

At first I said no to the surgery on those grounds. But it was my mother, the conventional beauty and choice feminist, who suggested I consider the surgery as an act of vanity, and vanity as a spectrum. There were many things we all did (and do) to take care of ourselves and "better" how we look: I wore braces; I obsessively cut and colored my hair (pink, then blue); I was maniacal, as all teenagers are, about my clothing (I'd call it proto-goth: lots of black, safety pins, and heavy on the eyeliner.) These were all somewhere on the spectrum. My mother asked me to consider at what end of the spectrum vanity encourages thoughtless superficiality, and at what end it encourages uplifting change. Smart mother. And while, at nearly eighteen, I did have a fairly raised consciousness, the truth is that I was also an unattractive girl who was tired of being unattractive. I chose the surgery and vowed not to apologize.

The surgery itself was supposed to be outpatient. I would be sedated with a local anesthetic and go home that evening. But I had an allergic reaction to the sedative and had to go under general anesthesia instead. When you have surgery on your face and you're breathing through a tube, all of the blood drains to your stomach. I was sick for days. The local anesthetic would have allowed me to remain awake throughout the procedure. The blessing of my allergy was that I slept through the smashing of my nose with an actual hammer, the gouging-out of the tumor, the scraping and chiseling and filing, the awkward reassembly. The recovery was excruciating. Between painkillers, my vision would blur and a pounding would erupt in my ears. I felt as if someone was embroidering an intricate pattern on the surface of my brain: There was a pattern of needle pricks, sometimes swirly, sometimes looping, but constant and overwhelming. I couldn't think; I didn't dream for weeks.

And I stayed in. I was swollen and bruised. My family called me "the Technicolor girl," as my face went from deep purple to glossy yellow to a dull, faint green. It was summer, and so I sat by the window fan, read, and watched TV. In the evenings I would walk through our leafy Detroit neighborhood with my father. I was almost eighteen, but I enjoyed holding his hand. And I loved his stupid jokes. ("Guess who I saw today?" "Who?" "Everybody I looked at!") We talked. He asked me questions about my future (Would I like to go to college, his college perhaps? Maybe I wanted to be a teacher or an architect or an actress. . . .). At the end of each walk, he would peel back the bandage and rave about how quickly I was healing. He called me strong and brave.

But character doesn't stand in for beauty, does it? As a girl, before the surgery, I was a gifted dancer, save for my nagging habit of looking down while onstage. It was a family joke that I would pay my way through college with the change I found while walking with my head down. I was careful never to turn sideways in front of a camera. I tried putting up pictures of Barbra Streisand—every big-nosed girl's idol—but it didn't help much. Yes, she was great in *Funny Girl* and *Funny Lady*, but she was no beauty—that was clear.

Once, when I was twelve, while my parents were out for the evening and my older brother and sister watched television, I locked myself in my parents' room and systematically destroyed every picture of myself that I could find. My parents came home to me asleep in the fetal position, my face puffy from crying. Around me was a lake of ruined photographs, each one punctured through the face.

A year after the bandages came off, in the year it took my new face to settle, I looked at myself in the mirror, and here is what I saw: a nineteen-year-old beauty with toasty-brown eyes that were huge, round, and clear, as well as lashy, set deep in Semitic circles and unblinking above broad, smooth, pink cheeks and geranium-red lips pulled back in a smile across straightened white teeth. And with an undistinguished, feminine nose with nostrils that didn't match each other. The whole face was framed by bouncy, shiny black hair. I stood back and assessed the rest: D cups, tiny waist, dancer's legs. . . . It all worked well together. I was pretty. "Lovely," my father would say, every time he got the chance to put his hand to my cheek and kiss the top of my head, "so lovely."

Once I was pretty, the predictable happened: I looked up. And I got a good look at how people looked at me. And it was that simple. My first night in the dorm at college, I was startled awake by my roommate, who said, "Listen." Outside, a herd of drunk upperclassmen was engaged in a rousing chorus of "Wake Up, Little Susie." Right then, I understood the possibilities of flirtation and of sex. The combination of nineteen years of cracking jokes and doing well in school and being pretty made my years in college and graduate school, and as a single woman in New York City, wild in the best possible way. I met and charmed a lot of people—women and men—and touched and tested and tasted and felt intimate and attractive and loved.

In graduate school, I experienced a defining moment when I met my friend Seth in a room full of other English Comp teaching assistants. We sat next to each other in the back, making sarcastic remarks about the dowdy lead instructor and cracking each other up. During a break in the instruction, he said to me, "You're way too funny for a pretty girl." Compliment accepted. I still wonder if pretty women who grew up as such are made to cultivate only their beauty. I wonder, too, if suddenly becoming pretty is preferable to always having been pretty, because in the becoming, there is room—demand, even—for so much else: wit, imagination, humor.

I'm relieved that I'll never know, never be, the woman who that big-nosed girl was going to be. I'm so glad that I interrupted her life and changed her face into this face, my face. I'm not sure who she would have grown up to be. Maybe someone sadder, quieter, with a less public job or a less social life. But I am sure she would have been a poet. That's the transformative beauty of writing. Anything felt can manifest as perfect. What you look like is precisely that—what you look *like*. And I know for certain that my losses would have been her losses. I started writing in earnest when my father was diagnosed with Alzheimer's disease during my third year of college. I had, until then, considered my identification with my beloved father—being *from* as well as *of* him—as the way in which I knew myself. When he began to fade, I had to replace him with another way of knowing and understanding, another way into myself. Writing balanced his leaving, and he would have left her too.

Ten years after the surgery, I was used to being pretty, maybe even a little bored with it, certainly not fulfilled by it. Physical beauty is moving but ultimately powerless. It reconciles nothing. And my own beauty took on a wicked irony when I was twenty-eight and my father died. I was the eulogist at his funeral, and his elegist in my poetry. I struggled to remember him, to memorialize him, and to claim, for always, my inheritance from him. So there was a time when I longed for that part of me that was a direct gift from him—that outward, awkward, front, forward, and center sign of Sephardic blood. There's some shame now in my missing nose. *Fixed, forgotten.*

From the time I was fifteen until my father had to give up his medical practice, he kept a framed photograph of me with my original nose on the wall above his desk. In the picture, my hair is greasy and matted to my head. I have on several heavy wool sweaters, and a compass and whistle hang from my neck. I am carrying a large backpack, which partly blocks the vista of bent, leafless trees and grim, gray sky. I am smiling triumphantly, as I have made it to the top of Silers Bald in the great Smoky Mountains. I am looking directly into the camera. When he put the photograph on display, I explained to my father that when the picture was taken, I had not seen a mirror in fourteen days. "I don't care," he said. "You look so beautiful." I keep that picture by my own desk now.

I am forty-two. I have been officially pretty longer than I haven't been. But now, when I look in the mirror, I'm sad to see my prettiness in retreat. I recall with a cringe the day I was busy running a live daily show on the public radio station where I worked, and some young man—still in college, but the kind of young man who would have wanted me, say, fifteen years before—called me "Ma'am." And he meant it—and not the way the college boys who tried to address me with respect when I taught Freshman Comp in graduate school meant it. I have stopped getting the pretty-girl discount, and it is taking an embarrassingly long time to get over that. Having not been pretty, then suddenly becoming pretty, then enjoying being pretty for two decades, then feeling the loss of my prettiness is to be full of arrogance and sorrow all at once.

In middle age, my hard-won babehood is something I have to lose. It's a true loss. I can't go on about this, though, because there is nothing worse than a pretty woman whining about the loss of her looks, particularly a pretty woman who has everything else: a healthy family, a thriving career, good-humored friends, a place to buy jeans that fit. I haven't yet found my way *through* the loss, either. I'm sad for the loss of my looks, and I'm ashamed of my sadness. I'm worried that this—twenty-two years later—*is* the feminist argument against plastic surgery:

Eventually, what you "had done" cannot undo the rest of the culture (which says that prettiness matters most); and that it can't undo nature (prettiness fades). I want to believe the uplifting idea that wisdom is a beauty all its own; that wrinkles give a face character; that gray hairs are just silvery highlights. I do believe, but mostly because it's silly not to.

Slowly I'm learning to let go of my pretty face. I'm learning to believe that prettiness matters less. My nose is just my nose; my face is just my face (and there's relief in that). This is what matters *more* than being pretty: I am an artist. And my art is significant to my work, and they are both about my craft—and that's a rare and beautiful thing. By "craft," I mean how I make my living. I do it by listening. I listen and pay attention. (No need for pretty. And as it turns out, I was born with a great set of ears.) My life is in sound; in breath and cadence and silence. My life is on the radio. My life is in that moment when you turn up the volume on your radio; when you close your eyes and open your ears and experience every possible person, place, taste, touch, sound, sign, and song there is. And my life is in poetry. I thought of the music of the human voice and the human voice in context, and put that music to paper, and I became a poet.

And this is what matters *most:* When I look at the beaming face of my seven-year-old daughter as she emerges from the swimming pool or her second-grade classroom, and I see that her big Jewish nose is already forming, I don't care. She is beautiful (of course), and she will be smart and funny, because we will help her cultivate her intelligence and her humor. And later, if she wants one, she can have a nose job.

ellen papazian
CONCEALER

The day my father couldn't take the concealer anymore is a day that is permanently seared into my brain. Twenty-four years later, I can replay the scene perfectly. I was sitting in his idling Mercedes outside his Stamford, Connecticut, apartment building—the one he fled to after leaving my mother. I was thirteen years old, and I had been deeply committed to concealer for about a year.

My father was already in a testy mood. It was after work on a Wednesday, the one day a week I saw him, and he had run into his apartment for something he'd forgotten. We were on our way to dinner at a Duchess fast-food restaurant. He was still in a business suit. I was in one of my outfits for school—way uncool non-Sasson jeans, a sleeveless sweater vest, and white socks with loafers, à la Michael Jackson. My father had just left the car when I habitually reached up to the passenger-side mirror and pulled it down to peer at my face, a concealer stick at the ready in my right hand.

My relationship with concealer started after my mother bought me the book *Scavullo Women*. Why a mother would buy her awkward, tall, bony, ugly-duckling twelve-year-old daughter—who was already cowering in one of the snobbiest counties in Connecticut—a large-format, glossy, four-color book celebrating world-renowned fashion photographer Francesco Scavullo's bevy of beauties is one for the mystery books. *Scavullo Women* was page after page of high-fashion photo spreads of models transformed from plain-looking, but still drop-dead gorgeous, to fully glammed-up and drop-dead gorgeous. Scavullo knew beauty. And he knew how to transform beauty into beauty. The first and most important step in this transformative process—I read with intent while secretively crouched in the attic of our house—was to use an excellent foundation and base on the model. Foundation was the cornerstone of a great work of art. Foundation was the make-up artist's most important tool. Foundation gave the artist a blank palette. It smoothed over every blemish, every line, and even dark circles under the eyes if a model stayed out too late or didn't drink her requisite regimen of water.

I studied the photos intently. The models were at their most beautiful in the "before" snapshots, when they were in their regular clothes, without makeup, but this, of course, wasn't the point. I marveled at their pretty features and skin. But the artist soon swooped in and smoothed over their skin his luscious foundation—making the model's face a perfect blank slate, with nary a bump, pimple, or mark. And it didn't stop there. After the lake of foundation, the make-up artist would add concealer under the model's eyes to remove any other imperfection or—*gasp*—dark circle. Patti Hansen, for instance, had dark circles. This is why concealer was the crucial final step to beautiful skin and a beautiful face.

I absentmindedly brought my hand to the half-moon shapes of skin underneath my eyes. I had dark circles. Yet they had nothing to do with lack of sleep. They had to do with the Armenians. My father's ancestors. The phenomenon of deep-set eyes: the defining feature of my not-yet-truly lived life. I would stand beside my mother as people met me and remarked upon me to her as if I weren't there.

"Oh, she looks different from you, Rita."

"Yes," said my mother, who was gorgeous, "she takes after her father."

"Ah, yes."

"She has his deep-set eyes."

"I see."

I studied the foundation-and-concealer stage of each Scavullo model makeover. And then I promptly went to Brooks Pharmacy and stole a Maybelline concealer. A tiny sheathed stick of sweet, pale perfection that fit snugly into the palm of my hand. I crouched in the aisle, took the concealer out of its package, slipped it into my tightened right fist, and exited the store, my heart pounding not just at my brazen act of lawlessness, but also at this newfound cure for my ugliness. I immediately went home, sat before the long, closet-door mirror in my bedroom, and carefully covered every part of my skin with concealer. I had stolen the palest option, and I watched how the place where my cheek normally shifted from petal pink to milky purple now became a stretch of pinkish-white, pasty landscape.

It took fifteen minutes of painstaking, sweeping hand movements before I became a blank palette of white skin, which I then topped off with black mascara and blush. I pulled my bangs off my face, secured them back with two barrettes, and combed out the long, stringy remainders of hair. I appraised myself in the mirror. And—it dumbfounds me even today— I did not think I looked pale. I thought I was closer to perfect. I thought I had a defense against anyone's piercing gaze. I could not be ugly if I did not have a blemish. I could not be ugly if I did not have one outstanding blip on the cast of my face.

The concealer regimen started to satisfy a deep longing inside of me. It became an internal conversation I had with myself about the art of being seen. It became my point of entry into the world. I could channel Scavullo. I could have just a tiny smidgen of Patti Hansen as I sat with my mother through her endless '80s disco parties with the community-newspaper journalist jet set. The parties were just one aspect of my mother's postdivorce Amazonian reawakening—her early-'80s revival of "I Am Woman, Hear Me Roar" that sometimes translated to "I Am Not Your Mother Right Now, Hear Me Roar" and left me bewildered in its wake. As I with my mother so often—caught in the headlights of her tiny, blue-eyed, determined stare—I felt a desperate need to erase the parts of myself that most resembled my father. Namely, the features of my face that were too large, too soft, and too Armenian. Sitting silently beside her in a bar booth at the parties, behind my freshly concealed face, I could be a white-sheathed antidote to her raven ringlets, wine-tipped fingernails, and blood-red Chanel lips. My concealment was not only my protection—it was my voice. *Just try to see the real me,* it called. *I am only what you think I am.* But in the light of the morning, sitting once again before the mirror with the concealer and sponge wedge in my hand, it also said, *Help me disappear.*

Or, *Disappear now.*

I followed my concealer beauty regimen every day. I even took to putting concealer on my lips—a bold move that I thought would further blend the many unseemly contours of my face—and no one remarked on the difference, until my father did.

He'd said nothing that day when he exited the car and I snatched the concealer out of my purse, ready to refresh my concealment. But he came back more suddenly than I had anticipated. I had cocked the rearview mirror to the passenger side and was midconcealment when he brusquely opened the door and started shouting at me.

"Goddammit, Ellen, will you *stop* putting that all over your face!"

He nearly pushed me off the gear shift and back to the passenger side. He yanked the rearview mirror back into place, cocked the Mercedes into reverse, and floored it out of the apartment driveway. I shoved the concealer back into my purse, my heart pounding with a thousand tiny embarrassments, and turned to watch the dull city streets flash by me on our way to Duchess.

My father had jerked me back to reality. I had thought the concealer would make me more beautiful, but I started to wonder if it was instead making me a freak. No one at school ever said anything, but then again, no one at school ever said I was pretty or—the unthinkable—sexy, or ever really asked me out.

The only times I had ever been kissed were planned moments—spin-the-bottle events that I happened to attend, or late-night hookups with boys I didn't know that usually took place at the beach, when I was nestled in the forgiving safety of darkness and they had no frame of reference for who I was, except that I was the friend of Claudine or Christina or Kim or any of the other well-endowed, doe-eyed, red-lipped girls who increased my boy-worthiness by 100 percent.

My father had made me feel like a freak and, in typical style, said nothing to make me feel otherwise. I yearned to say to him, "Dad, if I don't use my concealer, everyone will see in cold daylight how ugly I am! You just don't *get* it, *do* you?!" But that would have required him to engage with me about something personal, which was way beyond his capabilities. He was too busy flooring his Mercedes when the light turned green.

My father had brought a sudden consciousness to my behavior. Yet it was a jarring and embarrassing consciousness. In that split second, when he intruded on me midconcealment, I felt as exposed as a threadbare T-shirt yanked midcycle from a washing machine to be hung out, soaking, to dry. I knew in that moment that I could no longer conceal without the full understanding that what I was doing was aberrant and, most important, not pretty. That it was a behavior unsanctified in the all-pretty-girls-go-to-heaven landscape of my life. I knew that my till-then secret regimen now left me at serious risk, that if my father had noticed it, it would simply be a matter of time before everyone—the school, the town, the boys I'd never kiss, and, of course, all the girls—would know too. I tucked that knowledge beneath one of my slight ribs and pretended I did not possess it. There were other things to focus on (namely, procuring better-looking sleeveless sweater vests), and there was too much at stake for me to abandon concealer. If I did, I would have to uncover my real face—the one people, including my mother, so often looked at blankly, as if I were a creature needing to be figured out. I decided that I had to recommit myself to the Scavullo fantasy. I had the magical idea that since only my father had said something to me about my abnormally concealed face, then only my father had noticed it. My reasoning was based on this one fact: No one else, not even my mother, had said anything about it to me before.

My mother had actually never talked to me about beauty. It was as if when it came to my becoming a woman, she did not know what to say. Or if she did know what to say, it was as if she did not have the time, need, or desire to say it. Any beauty instruction from my mother that I encountered pre-Scavullo and pre-concealer was through osmosis. As a girl, I would stand beside her while she made herself pretty in the mirror, and then, after she left, I would let the heavy faux-gold Estée Lauder lipstick case weigh down my small hand, let it seep its wordless wisdom into me. By the time I was twelve, I felt so invisible that I didn't think I deserved instruction. I wouldn't make it onto the all-star beauty team, I reasoned, so why would it matter? I couldn't compete (the Armenian bone structure was all wrong), so I never bothered trying out. Yet what I was left with still felt unbearable, just as unbearable as walking by groups of girls or boys, or walking into class when everyone was already seated, or having to participate in rope climbing in the gym. I always felt like I had to hide. I felt like there was a gigantic gaze that told me I was ugly, and that the gaze kept finding new places to be.

So I continued to conceal, despite my father's outburst. I would conceal during all breaks between classes at Tomlinson Junior High, and I would conceal before I entered the cafeteria, the most frightening part of my day. I would conceal before I left school for home. I was always in the girls' bathroom, and I would put myself in harm's way to conceal. I was there so much that every burnout would negotiate every toke in my presence, and every frightening bully would freak out against the bathroom walls or in the stalls while I stood—in my baggy jeans and ever-present sweater vest—with a stick of concealer in my hand.

I remember one particular bully named Becky who, at fourteen, was rumored to be a mom already and was close to house arrest. She was yelling as she entered the bathroom after nearly tearing the face off of some girl in the hallway. She came pounding in (five times my size, without exaggeration), stomped into the stall behind me, and slammed its door shut. *"Fucking asshole motherfuckin' bitch!"* she screamed. She slammed the door so hard, it bounced open and shut again, the sound reverberating all throughout the bathroom. I noticed that her hair had changed color (from mousy brown to burnt sienna) and that her denim jeans were so thin, they seemed to be painted all over her wide hips and thighs.

"Fuckyoufuckyoufuckyoufuckyoufuckyou!"

I grasped the concealer and froze with it beneath my eye. I thought for a second that she might kill me, and decided to abandon the regimen. She came out of the stall and looked at me.

"Do you smoke?" she asked.

"No," I stammered. "Not yet," I added. (Perhaps the promise that I would be smoking soon would spare me?)

She stood still for a second and looked at me. She kept watching me as I lowered my head, put the concealer back into my makeup bag, and zipped it up in my LeSportsac. I prayed she wouldn't ask me for anything else, and I also felt this pressure inside my chest to figure her out, to ask her what no one dared to ask: *Do you have a child?*

But her voice interrupted my train of thought.

"What was that?" she challenged.

"What?" I asked.

"That," she said, "in your hand."

"It's concealer," I said. "It corrects blemishes and dark circles on your face." I don't know why I felt the need to explain this to her. Everyone knew makeup by the time they got to Tomlinson.

"I want it," she said.

She stared at me.

I knew she didn't really want my concealer. I knew she just wanted to play a game of psychological warfare with me, but I gave it to her. It was a matter of survival. I reasoned that because she had a child, Becky had a lot to deal with already, and she probably did not have the money to get concealer (though no money was needed, since I stole mine), and what's more, she probably needed something to lift her spirits in her harsh, smoke-filled, F-word–laden world. I felt better thinking that it was good to bow down to Becky. And I also felt a flicker of lightness in the split-second moment when I let my concealer slip out of my hand and into hers. She stalked away from me, turned at the swinging door, and heaved her enormous back against it, opening it with her body. She did it so freely—keeping her solid gaze set on mine—that I felt a shift in the floor beneath me. I held my breath and watched the edges of her burnt-sienna hair chisel into the stale hallway air.

The concealer stick itself was cheap and flimsy—each phallic, plastic case so battered around in my makeup bag that it became brittle and chipped, with its artificial skin tone rubbed to dull white. Yet in the bathroom with Becky, feeling the concealer leave my hand, I realized that it had a weight beyond its weight, a matter within its own matter—a currency to exchange.

I imagined how Becky would transform herself now that she possessed my concealer stick. I pictured her morphing into a subtler, more feminine version of herself—more Olivia Newton-John than Meatloaf. *Would she become more distant from the world, and from her anger, thanks to the intrinsic power of the concealer stick? Was Becky's child a girl or a boy? Who took care of it?*

Also: *Was Becky pretty when she had sex for the first time?* The shiny teen magazines that had drifted down to me—all of them snakeskin sheddings of *Scavullo Women*—promised that we'd be pretty when we did it, after gorging ourselves on make-up tips and lying around, waiting for the boys. *What was it like when Becky did it? Was she pretty when she did it, or was she invisible, hidden in a dark backroom closet inside a tiny home?*

I looked into the mirror. I was hidden. And I also wanted to know: *Would I be hidden when I did it, beneath the thick lake of liquid, paste, and powder?*

*By age fourteen I had discovered concealer powder, in beau-*tiful, turquoise oval containers, and glass-bottled foundation, akin to liquid gold. I inherited my mother's older bottles of Estée Lauder foundation, so wet they practically leaked from the glass as they sat upon my shelf. They sweated promise, but they were also so thin and liquidy that I could not expertly apply them to my face. And they were also not the palest white shade I was used to procuring on my theft outings, so I often was stuck with a two-toned face. Patchy and dark and pasty and white.

I didn't notice all the snafus I made with the liquid gold and the concealment stick until I saw a photograph taken by a lake during a rare nature hike with my dad. I was wearing a long-sleeved black shirt, which didn't help matters, and I was also smiling widely with my braces (another beauty faux pas), but the midday sun beating down on my face highlighted the truth: I looked like a patchy ghost. There was nothing smooth about my skin, no beautiful palette. I was a Scavullo failure—and an awkward and insecure girl on top of it.

Despite the fact that I hated the lakeside photo, I taped it into my journal and wrote beneath it, "Me, 1984." Looking at it, I would feel a deep sense of regret about my looks, but I also left it where it was taped and continue to write away my days—dreaming of future kisses, groundbreaking love, and success as a professional photographer. I did not dream of modeling or being anywhere in front of a camera. I dreamed about being behind one.

One night, after my father's outburst about the concealer, my friend Kim—one of those blessed skinny girls with boobs and full lips—came to my house to sleep over, and I showed her the Scavullo book. I didn't show it to many people, and I never, ever let my mother see me read it. I kept it on my shelf next to the biography of Diane Arbus and the old, dog-eared *World of Pooh*. I still felt that I was in communion with the secret of beauty when I opened it up and inhaled the sleek smell of perfection and sex and grace. I took it off the shelf and handed it to Kim without really thinking and said to her, "Look at the models in here. It tells you how to do your makeup, too."

She grabbed the book and turned through all the pages in about ten minutes before saying to me, "Let's make ourselves over."

"Okay," I said.

I was beginning to feel a little wary of the task, but still, I was game.

"And let's do it by putting on as much makeup as we can. I mean gobs of it," she added.

She asked where my makeup was, and I showed her the hand-me-down basket of wares my mother had given me, and then I opened my bag of tricks: concealer sticks, foundation bottles, and pancake cases with moist, flat pads. She rifled through it with an insouciance that I associated only with Madonna. Then we washed up and retired to the den in front of the TV, where we unloaded all the makeup in the center of the room and went to town on each other's faces. I concealed and concealed and concealed till she laughed so much that tears ran deep rivers of pancake into her cheeks. She slathered me with liquid rouge and lipstick layers, but refused to use any concealer. I felt totally naked yet filled with a sense of enormity. I felt as if the self inside my body—the one so familiar to me as small—was doubling every second, like I had sixteen Beckys pushing out from inside.

It took us about two hours to do each other's faces. The rule was, you could not see the finished product until it was done. Kim went first. I took her into the bathroom, and she was giggling even before she looked, but when she saw her face—bizarre and truly ghastly—she burst into laughter. Already the eye-pencil lines and mascara layers had dripped down her cheeks, and the foundation was so thick and outrageous that even *I* couldn't stand it. I wanted to get the washcloth right away. Then Kim put me in front of the mirror, and I saw, for the first time, things about my face I hadn't seen in nearly two years: how my eyes settled into the half-moon circles beneath them, and how a slight gold dusted the hazel. I also saw the theater that was me: the layers of mauve and lines of charcoal that did nothing but create more distance between me and the world that waited for me.

We couldn't wait to take the makeup off. We did so feverishly. My skin was pulsing in the air. We stayed up way past *Saturday Night Live* and then crashed in my bedroom on the second floor. We kept the windows half-cracked, and as a car passed by outside and spun its lights along my ceiling, Kim asked me why on earth we had to care about makeup at all—why we felt we had to make ourselves look pretty.

"I don't know," I said. "But it's *sooooo* annoying."

"I know," she said. "It's completely stupid, too."

Easy for her to say, I thought. *She's pretty.* But I knew by then I had to agree. "It *is* stupid."

The next morning, after Kim left the house, I sat before the closet-door mirror and started my routine. I took the concealer stick out of my bag and picked up the sponge wedge with my other hand. I leaned into the mirror and focused on the purple circles beneath my eyes, but then I stopped. I felt a new presence in my mind, a change. I had the sudden realization that Kim was, quite possibly, a teenage medicine woman. And that by slathering and slathering the makeup on me, she had also—with her fast-working hands—whipped from my true face the hundreds of fake concealer faces I had painted on before. It was as if they had all been crepe-paper faces, disintegrating in her hands before they even reached the floor.

I pictured my crepe-paper faces and Kim's fast-moving hands. I pictured Kim's face when I brought her to the bathroom mirror—when I stood behind her and held her bony shoulders with my sweaty palms, and she looked into the mirror at the theater of a face that was not hers and, without wasting a beat, broke it apart with her giant laugh. I remembered the way her laugh made her face fall into itself—made her fake face fall into her real face, and made her real face emerge again: alive, breathing. I remembered my own face. It seemed important to let it live, too. I looked at the stick and put it back in the makeup bag. I zipped up the bag, opened the closet door, and threw it onto the floor. Then I took the Scavullo book off the shelf and went upstairs to the attic, where we kept all our old books. We each had our own box. I tossed it in mine.

My father never mentioned anything to me about my concealer-free face. We still had our Wednesday dinners, and we played lots of Ms. Pac Man while waiting at Duchess for our hamburgers. I got good at Ms. Pac Man. I loved the thrill of being chased by the blue ghosts while striving for the cherry. I loved the sound it made when I ate that cherry right up. Each stage of the game I got through, my heartbeat kicked my mind into gear, and I focused on the next stage and set myself on winning. I was so anxious in between the stages, I nearly paced in place at the machine. But when the screen went blank, I saw my face looking back at me in the darkened space. I could see how my features—the nose that had seemed too large, the teeth too protruding, and the eyes too deeply set—were no longer placid, but electric and elastic. They were neither pretty nor ugly, but simply present. They slid quickly, almost wildly, into shapes that signaled that I was a person completely engaged. No longer part of the disappeared, but part of the alive. My features created the necessary, now sparkling, pattern of my face. It was the face of a player. The face of a seeker in the uncharted terrain of my adolescent life. Even in that split second, I could see the many ways the screen captured the whole truth of my face before unleashing it back to the game.

kristen buckley
WHAT I AM IS WHAT I AM

Not long ago I was in Hawaii, staying in an exclusive four-star hotel with my children. The place was teeming with people from Los Angeles (Hollywood types have a bad habit of vacationing in all the same places), and I noticed that my kids recognized a few other kids from their local park. Each day, I'd take them to the hotel pool, and they would play with these children while the mothers congregated on the opposite side of the pool. They did not speak to me or acknowledge me, other than with a curt hello. I didn't really think much of it and happily read my magazines. When I returned to L.A., my children's nanny told me that those women thought I was a new nanny, which was why they didn't interact with me.

A few months later, I was having lunch at the Bel Air Hotel. On the way out, I went into the bathroom to wash my hands, and a smartly dressed woman in her late thirties turned to me rather gruffly and muttered, "You need to put more toilet paper in there."

These aren't isolated incidents for me. I have had clothes handed to me at a Laundromat. I have been given documentation at the DMV that is exclusively in Spanish. I have been asked not to loiter. During some lean years I spent waiting tables at the White Horse Tavern, a half-drunk customer said to me, "What kind of Negro are you, anyway?"

In the moment, I rarely realize what's going on. Usually I'm just confused. When the woman at the Bel Air Hotel told me about the toilet paper, I assumed she was giving me a heads-up. When the man at the Laundromat handed me his clothes, I thought it was because he needed help. It's only later that I realize these people were expecting me to serve them. It's then that their presumption of superiority gets to me. It burrows in and makes itself at home deep inside my bones. It whispers to me when I am tired (or down, or facing a tough time) that my life might be easier (or better, or richer) if I just had blond hair and blue eyes. Hearing this whisper makes me angry, not because I want a different life, but because I'm tired of being judged unfairly because of my face. Yet I have nowhere to air my grievances.

In America, the way you identify your racial heritage is often a source of commonality among people. Our own Census Bureau frames instructions on ancestry in a manner that discourages the response "multiple." You are expected to be able to reveal a precise historical identity. But I cannot.

I am a mutt, a conflation of Celtic, Mediterranean, and northern African. I can say with certainty that my mother is

Irish, which makes me half Irish, though you'd never know it from looking at me. As my mother says, "There's not a single girl in Ireland with your face," which is true, because my face is my father's. My nose is a bit wide; my eyes are deep-set; I have high cheekbones and an enormous forehead, all framed by a mass of curly dark hair that I lighten. It is odd to look in the mirror and see the face of your estranged father—the one who left you, the one you don't speak to. It is, in some ways, like living with a ghost.

Where did this ghost face of mine come from? That is a more difficult question. My father's ancestry is clouded in mystery. If you look at my father, and his sisters and his mother, you can't help but see African features, despite the light skin. There were rumors that my father's grandmother, the red-haired tutor from Spain who may have been crazy or cruel, was the mistress of my great-grandfather, who was either a mysterious dark-skinned Tunisian or an African real estate tycoon, or both. Or neither. It depends on whom you talk to. Long ago, before we stopped speaking, I asked my father if we were part black, and he said we were. But he has since rescinded that, and now any mention of it is met with blatant hostility. I suspect this is because my father now lives in the Deep South, a place still influenced by the absurdity of the "one drop" rule, where talk of African blood only creates problems.

In truth, I don't even know what word to use to describe myself. "Biracial" isn't right. "Multiethnic" seems vague. The Oxford English Dictionary describes a person having one-eighth black blood (i.e., one black great-grandparent) as an octoroon. Somehow I don't think this description will go over well at dinner parties. I wish I could see a photograph of my great-grandfather, who may or may not have been black. There were no photos of him, at least none that I ever saw, and this has only deepened the mystery regarding my own face. I do not look particularly European; I certainly do not look Scandinavian; I don't look Celtic. But I do know that if I had lived in South Africa during the apartheid years, I would have been subjected to a Pencil Test, and I would have failed. (For the unfamiliar, South Africa devised a delightfully simple way to ascertain black blood. If you placed a pencil in a person's hair and it fell out, that person was classified as white. If it remained in, the person was "colored." By their standards—and the three pencils currently stranded in my hair—I'm definitely "colored.")

There is no multiethnic task force representing those who cannot be lumped into a particular group. There's no Quasi-Rainbow Coalition. No National Association for the Advancement of People Who Might Be Colored but Whose Families Are Sort of Crazy and Won't Talk About Their Ethnic Background Because They Have Issues. I don't see many people who look like me. I don't know anyone who has a background like mine. I may live in Southern California, but I reside inside a multiethnic no-man's land. I am too light to complain, and too dark to fit in. I'm convinced that this is why, when people learn about my work as a successful screenwriter and novelist, when they Google my name, or even when they meet my children, they express amazement at my accomplishments. I know this isn't because my eight-year-old daughter understands three languages or because my five-year-old is a whiz at baseball. It's because they have low expectations of me based on the way I look.

The other day, I caught a glimpse of myself in a mirror at the Banana Republic in Beverly Hills. For a brief moment I was caught by surprise by the quirky, bohemian-looking woman I saw there. She looked interesting and different—like someone I'd like to meet. Then I realized she was me, and it got me thinking: What if my face has been the largest factor shaping my life? More than my upbringing, more than my education, more than my childhood traumas and my mistakes and sins of commission and omission . . . what if *it* alone has shaped my life?

I considered the facts that might bolster this theory: The burden of a confused identity forced me to confront who I was early on. Because I did not live in a multiethnic community, I had no place of refuge. Without refuge, I never became beholden to any particular group. I was never forced to check off a single box to which I had to conform. Because of this, my thoughts, from an early age, were not shaped by social constraints and expectations; they were shaped by self-direction and autonomy. My face has allowed me to roam—like a nomad—and experience a world of possibilities that might not be available to someone on the inside.

So while I have always lived with a certain degree of alienation, and I am occasionally mistaken for "the help," it may be that this is just a karmic reality of having a face without borders—a face that represents a confluence of places and people and time and geography. It is a face like no one else's, and maybe this is what has allowed for the creative life I lead. When I'm not being mistaken for the help, people tend to label me as "groovy" or "interesting," sometimes even "kooky" or "wacky." And maybe I am all of those things. With a face like mine, no one questions why I have a younger boyfriend, or how it is that I send my daughter to French school, even though I don't speak a word of the language myself. A face like this gives me permission to get a tattoo in ancient Greek on my arm, or to start an online magazine with my best friend, train for a 5k, or even write romantic comedies.

My face gives me freedom. Its uniqueness represents my own personal geography. And maybe people want to define it because they are used to living inside boundaries drawn on maps, whereas I live in a country where there are no boundaries.

louise desalvo

FACELESS

1.

In the tenement on Adams Street in Hoboken, New Jersey, from my cot in the room that I share with my parents, I can see, tucked into a corner of the mirror, a holy picture of Jesus Christ on the cross.

The picture is small. Just a few inches wide, a few inches tall. I am a child, and each time I look to the mirror, what I see terrifies me. It's not my face I see—my attention is drawn to the Crucifixion. A man in pain beyond comprehension. A man unable to hold his head upright, the inclined head alone an account of suffering incarnate. A head with matted hair. A head crowned with thorns. The thorns puncturing the flesh, bloody rivulets running down the face. The hands punctured too and oozing blood, for—as my mother has told me when I have asked—nails have been pounded through his body. And

I can see the nails, the stab wounds in the torso. Feet nailed to the cross. Blood, blood, and more blood.

I am two years old, then three, then four, then five—and tall enough to see into the mirror when I stand on the floor—then six, then seven. And through those years, the mirror is not something I want to look into, to see my face, to primp before, to ascertain how my visage has changed, to see how I've grown. The mirror is not something I use, as my playmate upstairs does, to make silly faces in front of, or to make sure that she is brushing her hair just so, or to see the results of a session of playing dress-up in her mother's clothes, imagining what she will look like as a woman grown. So when I'm seven, and we move from the tenement in Hoboken to the house in Ridgefield, New Jersey, I have not developed the habit, as other girls do, of looking at myself to primp, of seeing who I am or who I might become, of wondering how others see me.

When my family moves into the house in Ridgefield, the mirror from the apartment gets moved into my parents' room. The holy picture disappears. My mother decorates our room. Patterned wallpaper with roses. Chenille bedspread. Sheer curtains. Comfy area rugs. My parents buy my sister and me a new mirror in a wooden frame for our bedroom. They hang it on the wall atop our dresser.

On the dresser, in front of the mirror but off to one side, my mother places a very large framed picture of Christ crucified, a giant version of the one from before. Same inclined head crowned with thorns, same matted hair, same punctured and ravaged flesh, same rivers of blood, same scene of suffering and torture as before—only much, much larger.

My mother has taken some care with this detail of our room's decor. She has shopped for it, she has measured it, she has had it framed, and she has placed it just so, so that every time my sister or I look into it, we will see it counterpoised against the image of our own faces. The image was horrifying to me then, and still is, for it shows me not how Christ suffered for the sins of man, but instead how brutal people can be, and how they can harm one another, and that the world is not a safe place for any of us.

Years later, when a friend from college enters my room and sees it—for it is still there—she asks, "What is this, Crucifixion Central?" And this is the first time I suspect that Christ crucified is not an altogether normal embellishment for the room of two girls. Now my mother is long dead, and I cannot ask her why she did this. But I do know that it wasn't because she was a deeply spiritual woman. There were times she went to church and times she didn't; times she took the sacraments and times she didn't.

Did my mother place this horrifying image before the mirror to ensure that we would spend no more time in front of the mirror than was absolutely necessary? Did she want to prevent my sister and me from becoming narcissistic mirror gazers, hair tossers, primpers, girls more interested in appearance than in character? Did she want to remind us that whatever difficulties we experienced—my father's rages, her depressions, our childhood sufferings—counted for little or nothing in the context of such enormous pain? Or, instead, was this to be a *memento mori*, a reminder of our mortality?

2.

The mirror is and always has been an anguished place. I spend time in front of it only when absolutely necessary: when I am a young girl, and my father tells me to get myself in front of the mirror to comb my disheveled hair *or else;* when, as an adolescent, I put on my makeup as quickly as I can.

As a teenager, I have the habit of standing in front of the mirror and looking at myself when I am crying, when I am enraged, or when I am terrified because my father is on one of his rampages. I have the habit of standing in front of the mirror and sticking my tongue out at myself in derision after my parents have told me that I have not done, yet again, what I was supposed to do. I have the habit of standing in front of the mirror to see if my last battle with my father has resulted in any bruises, and to determine whether I will have to wear, yet again, a high-necked, long-sleeved shirt to school instead of the V-neck sweater I love.

Most times, though, I avoid looking into the mirror. For when I do, I see the image of myself juxtaposed with that of Christ crucified.

3.

That portrait of Christ, as I think of it now, denied me a sense of my own image; it denied me the ability to look at myself and see who I was, who I was becoming.

But it also denied me a sense of the reality and extremity of my own pain as a child and as a young woman, for whatever I suffered seemed so much less than that suffering. Reflected back to me as I witnessed myself crying, or enraged, or terrified, or harmed, was only a simulacrum of greater suffering. Whatever anguish or pain I felt, however harmed I was, it did not count. My pain could not compare with an anguish far greater than any I could ever experience.

4.

And yet.

There was my father's violence. Always, my father's violence. Unpredictable. Coming without any reason, at least to me. He hit me. Came at me with a knife. Choked me. Tried to smother me. But even more fearsome were his threats of violence greater than what I'd already experienced.

I'll break every bone in your body.

The next time you do that, I promise that I will kill you.

If I get my hands on you, I'll break your neck.

If you say that one more time, I'll rip your arm off.

If I catch you, I'll throw you out the window.

Though I did not know it at the time, the image of Christ crucified represented to me my father's brutality. It reminded me, every time I looked in the mirror, that I was not safe. I did not learn that the body can be cherished by those we love. That the people we love can be kind to us. I learned that the body can be harmed, and that being wounded is the natural order of things. And my mirror—reflecting back bruises, tears, scratches— told me this more often than I care now to remember.

5.

And there was this, too.

I believe that my mother's attachment to the image of Christ crucified, and her insistence on its being placed where we couldn't avoid seeing it, represented her own internal suffering. Hers was a primal and deep sorrow that overwhelmed our family. When it overcame her during summers—and she could barely clothe herself, barely shove something inedible in front of us at mealtimes, barely tend to a lacerated knee from our unsupervised, tempestuous play—my sister and I would be sent away to relatives. If it came on during the school year, we did the best we could without her care, walking to school in the rain without boots or umbrellas, eating frozen turkey dinners barely defrosted, wearing our underwear outside in, then inside out, day after day after day.

There was no way for my mother to name what came upon her. No way for her to tell us where she vanished to during these times. No way for her to comprehend why ordinary life distressed her. And so perhaps this image was meant to tell us, in a way that she could not, what the essence of her agony looked like. To look in the mirror, to see Christ's image before it, was to see my mother's suffering incarnate.

6.

When my mother was about ten months old, her mother died from influenza during the great epidemic. After her mother died, my mother stopped eating and almost died.

Her father, who had to travel to upstate New York for his work on the railroad, placed her with relatives. She began to gain weight slowly and was soon out of danger. Then her care became an imposition, and her relatives refused to continue what had become a burden to them; caring for their own children was difficult enough. My grandfather found another woman to care for her, but she was neglected, and the money was siphoned off to feed and clothe the woman's own children. When my grandfather came to see my mother unexpectedly, he found that she was starving.

One caregiver followed another until he found a job on the docks in New York City and sent for a woman in his native province of Puglia to marry him and to care for his daughter. This woman, though, could not love my mother, and whatever care she got was roughly and disinterestedly provided. My mother survived. That is, she survived corporeally. But even as a young child, she became so depressed that she was institutionalized and given shock treatments. I learned all of this after she died; while my mother is alive, she never speaks of her birth mother, never tells my sister or me how she almost died, never tells us the story. Of her suffering and sorrow.

7.

In the moving pictures of my mother and me when I am a child, she never looks at me. There are no moments when she gazes into my eyes. No pictures of her looking at me while she combs my hair. None of her smiling at me while I play dress-up or as we bake together. I have learned, from a book called *No Voice Is Ever Wholly Lost*, by Louise Kaplan, that the loving gaze of a mother or caregiver is incorporated into self-love. The mother's gaze: the first mirror of the self.

Why could my mother not look at me? Was it because she was so depressed, so locked into herself, that she did not have the emotional energy for a child? Or was it instead that looking into my face was too painful for her?

One day, when sorting through memorabilia my father gave me after my mother's death, I find two large and crumbling wedding photographs. One of my grandfather and the woman I have come to know as my grandmother. And one of my grandfather and my mother's birth mother. I have never seen this photograph before, never seen what my birth grandmother looked like.

I take it into my bedroom. Prop it up in front of my mirror. Look at her. Look at myself.

I am in my late forties, more than twenty years older than she was when she died. Still, there is a stunning resemblance between us. My face looks like what hers would have looked like had she grown as old as I am now.

Was it that my mother could not look at me because I reminded her of her dead mother? Was my face a too-painful embodiment of her loss? Or was it that her caregivers did not look at her, and so she never learned how to gaze at a child? But no, for there are many pictures of my mother looking at my sister. I know that I am the one she could not look at. I am the one she could not bear to see. And if my mother never looked at me, is it any wonder that I cannot see myself?

8.

In 1972, when I am thirty years old, I embark upon a series of paintings of faceless women. The first ones are of a single woman, in stylized dress, against a bold ground of color. The next are abstractions of mothers who embrace children yet are indifferent to them. Next are groups of three women, each detached from the others. Always, the women are faceless. And always, they seem sorrowful.

Back then, when I was asked why I painted women in this way, I said I wasn't interested in the specific features of a woman's face. I said I was interested only in portraying archetypal women. I could not have said that I was painting faceless women because of the faceless women in my life. My mother, who had disappeared into the facelessness of despair. Her birth mother, who had been erased from our family's history. And perhaps even the painter herself, who did not have the habit of looking at herself in the mirror.

9.

At more than sixty years of age now, I could not tell you what I look like, could not say how my face has changed or stayed the same throughout the years, could not say whether I consider myself beautiful, or plain, though some (but never my parents) have said that I am beautiful. (My mother's and my father's words: *Beauty is as beauty does.)*

Until I am in my fifties, I do not even know the color of my eyes.

Once, I have to indicate this detail, the color of my eyes, on a form. I go into the bathroom to look in the mirror to learn, for the first time, their color. Greenish-brown—what some call hazel—and rimmed with black. The same as my mother's. Or so my father has told me.

Can a woman spend her adult life combing her hair, putting on makeup—foundation, eyeliner, eye shadow, mascara, blush, lipstick (some of which I use each day)—and not know what she looks like? I see skin that is being covered with foundation. The eye outlined. The cheek taking on the color of the rouge. The shape of the lip turning red. I see all these things. But I do not see myself.

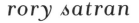

rory satran

NOT KNOWING

I took pictures of myself. And posted them on the Internet. There. I admit it.

"What's the big deal?" you might ask. "Why do you feel like you have to out yourself?" A cursory tour of Facebook or MySpace (I am a member of both) reveals the extent of the trend. Everyone's doing it. Preteens, teens, and adults alike are posing under perfect lighting in their bedrooms, the outstretched arm at the edge of the frame revealing their solitude. A recent *New York Times* article by Alex Williams dubbed these ubiquitous self-portraits "a kind of folk art for the digital age."

So where is the harm? Why the shame?

I was recently on a roller coaster at an amusement park. A teenager seated in front of me spent the entire ride with a digital camera in his hand, recording his own reactions as we hurtled through the air. At the end of the ride, he eagerly pressed play and watched himself live through the experience once again. This is the kind of thing I'm afraid of: being robbed of an experience for the sake of recording it. Not being able to live in the moment because I'm too concerned with the button to be pressed, the tilt of my head. Looking into the camera instead of at the world around me.

And therein lies the harm. And the shame is for an overdose of good old-fashioned narcissism. Everyone knows the deal. We are not supposed to be overly interested in our own image, because it prevents us from being interested in other people and things. Ovid's tale is the story of a man, Narcissus, who wilted away on the banks of Echo Pond because he was so completely enraptured by his own appearance. It should be a clarion call to my generation. Never has an entire generation of young people been so engrossed in snapping endless pictures of themselves, and posting them online for all the world to see. It's a new breed of narcissism—a narcissism of the digital age.

I am not at the level of Narcissus, or even Roller Coaster Boy. I am not one of those MySpace photo whores who sets a backdrop, turns up the volume on iTunes, and vogues away in front of my Canon Elph. I joined MySpace and Facebook after college, when I moved to Paris, simply because I wanted to keep in touch with my friends back home.

Before I joined these online communities, taking a self-portrait never would have occurred to me. Honestly. What would I have done with it? But as I delved deeper and deeper into the recesses of these sites, I was faced with lovely, but calculated, photographs of friends, friends of friends, and friends of friends of friends. Pictures of people with smooth hair, just-so smiles, and stylish clothing. Quite the opposite of my personal photo collection, which mainly comprised shots my dad took every year at six o'clock on Christmas morning. In these pictures I'm typically wearing my pajamas and glaring at the camera, my hair puffed up around my head like Krusty the Clown.

As I spent time browsing the profiles of others, I came across one girl in particular who caught my interest. A friend of a friend whom I had never met: I'll call her Miss X. Miss X's Facebook and MySpace pages were punctuated with some of the loveliest pictures I'd ever seen outside of a fashion magazine. Black-and-white nouvelle vague marvels in which Miss X's bangs are combed perfectly across her forehead, her eyes twinkling mysteriously at the camera. Miss X in stunning, eccentric outfits. In one particular shot that I started to obsess about, she's perched daintily on a pool table in a ruffled dress, holding the cue at a seductive angle. Her other arm holds the camera. It appears that every photo Miss X takes is a self-portrait.

Suddenly I, too, wanted to put pretty pictures of myself on the Internet. Pictures that captured my hair the way it was right after I brushed it, that kindly ignored the lower half of my body, that squinted forgivingly at my profusion of freckles. Basically, I wanted to capture the best version of myself. That fleeting moment when everything looks just right. The way I feel when I'm walking in the sunshine in my favorite jeans. And it seemed that I was the only person who could take such a picture. I'm not Lindsay Lohan; paparazzi don't follow me down the street.

My friends were sick of logging on to my homepage and seeing a big question mark in the space where my profile photo should have been. They weren't the impetus behind my new-found hobby, but I was getting plenty of encouragement to start clicking away. When I unexpectedly received a digital camera for Christmas that year, it was the incentive I needed to begin my shameful solitary photo shoot. I could finally foray into the mirrored funhouse of Miss X and the other girls and boys who controlled and played with their Internet images. I too would inspire cyber-admirers to leave rhapsodic comments on my web pages.

I planned my first photo session like a Russian mail-order bride preparing her online profile. I had to wait until my live-in boyfriend left, of course. I was too embarrassed to tell him what I was doing. I decided to set the manual timer on my camera instead of holding it out in front of my face. It seemed like a baby step toward my venture into self-portraiture, since I was far from ready to flaunt the telltale arm on the side of the frame that boasts: *I took this myself, and I don't care!* It was important to me that the picture look like it was taken by someone else. I wanted to avoid the extreme pout, the artificial background, the forced accessories.

But, I wondered, what exactly did I want to convey in this picture that would soon become public property, circulated and devoured by both friends and total strangers on the Internet? I wanted to depart from my usual style—hair in a bun (dubbed the "nun-do" by my best friend in sixth grade), no makeup, jeans, and a striped T-shirt. That is my everyday self, the girl who gets carded for R-rated movies at age twenty-four. I wanted to appear different from her, but how? Certainly I wouldn't pose on a pool table in a flouncy dress. I may have appreciated Miss

X's photos, but that wasn't me. Sure, I wanted to capture some of her style and fantasy, but I also wanted to retain my own essence. The problem was, I wasn't exactly sure what my essence was. I found myself frozen with doubt. A simple self-portrait had thrown my entire self-perception into question.

I tried on a navy blue polka-dotted T-shirt and a pair of jeans. Pulled my hair out of its nun-do and let it curl around my shoulders. Then I put on lipstick, something I rarely do in real life. In first grade, I convinced my mother to let me wear lipstick for my class picture. I fully assumed that when I was older I would look like Dolly Parton in *9 to 5*: full makeup, cleavage, and high heels. Now that I'm here, I look more like Lily Tomlin in the same flick. On her day off. That early childhood obsession with all things pink, sparkly, and artificial faded not too long after that first-grade photo shoot. I prefer a natural, classic look, and I have for quite some time. So as I smeared on bright lipstick, I felt as though I was regressing to the girlie-girl I'd abandoned long ago, the little girl who ran toward the spotlight, rather than shrinking from it.

I switched on the lamps in my apartment to create a soft glow. I arranged my camera on the coffee table. I peered through the viewfinder, picking out the spot where I would sit cross-legged on the floor. And I pressed the time-release button and ran backward and got into a sitting position, arranging my features into what I thought was an attractive expression, as the red light flashed patiently. Needless to say, the shot was far from great. There I am, peering expectantly at the camera with a frightened look. I found the whole process terribly embarrassing. I found myself wondering how Miss X managed to look so confident and sexy. Didn't it feel odd to play with fake emotions with no one else around to take the piss out of you? I looked around my apartment nervously, as though God was watching me and rolling his eyes. I closed the curtains. And tried again. And again.

The thing about digital cameras is that you can erase and retake pictures to your heart's content, particularly when you are all alone and there is no one there to guffaw at your vanity. If your left elbow looks chubby, or your skin too sallow, it's erased forever with a simple click. Which is all very nice. The danger for perfectionist types like me is that the picture will never be right. The cycle is endless: Pose. Flash. Erase. Repeat.

I became like Narcissus at Echo Pond; the hours melted away. I was obsessed with getting the perfect picture, one in which my chin looked shorter, my lips plumper, my cheeks fresher. In short, a picture in which I looked less like myself and more like an idealized version of myself.

That first photo shoot lasted far too long; afterward, I whittled down the endless images to two or three. I posted what I considered the best one of these on my Facebook and MySpace profiles. It was blurred. I had moved at the last minute, and my features were indistinct. All you could see was my long hair, my pink lips, and the polka dots of my shirt. There were other, clearer portraits, but I was aiming for fantasy, as opposed to reality. Ultimately, I realized I was too uncomfortable to go all out with my online self-portrait. I learned that I am a somewhat mediocre exhibitionist.

The lipstick and the flowing hair weren't the only uncharacteristic elements of those first self-portraits. I also found that

I adopted an almost angry-looking, sulky expression—a more extreme version of Miss X's knowing pout. I prefer the way my face looks when it's controlled, snobbish, and cold. This is odd, considering my naturally silly and smiling state. A typical photo of me (taken by someone else) invariably features me with crossed eyes and a goofy laugh. I suppose I saw my self-portraits as a way to counter the clownish image that I had been projecting for so long. Posing for myself gave me the opportunity to be the kind of reserved and mysterious woman I envy. I have always felt the need to be overly garrulous, worrying that people won't like me if I am too quiet, that I will disappear if I ever shut up. I have never been confident that others will seek me out of their own accord, without energetic prompting on my part. In those serious pictures I took in the privacy of my little apartment, I became that sphinxlike girl who attracted attention without asking for it.

The pictures I took that evening reveal a fantasy version of me: a cooler, more polished variation on my outgoing, natural self. But the fact is that I don't have the time or the inclination to be that woman in my everyday life. I don't want to bother to apply makeup in the morning, nor do I want the extra attention I'm sure would come along with it. I feel comfortable with my nun-do. And I may aspire to be more aloof and less forthcoming, but ultimately, that's just not me.

I still cringe over the memory of that first photo shoot, even though I've long since erased the evidence from my MySpace account. For the scant few weeks that that image represented me online, no one commented on it on my personal message board—except for my brother, who noted that it was blurry. It wasn't exceptional to anyone else that I was wearing lipstick, or that my hair was loose, my face holding an icy expression.

After I erased the self-portrait, I went back to the question mark. Since I wasn't sure what image I wanted to project into the wilds of the Internet, the anonymous blue question mark seemed newly profound. I don't necessarily want to look like an airbrushed fantasy, nor do I want to immortalize myself in my average nun-do authenticity. The question mark will work until I have a new idea of what I want to look like. And after all, isn't *not* knowing what my early twenties are supposed to be all about?

Not long ago, I finally met Miss X in the flesh through the friend we have in common. She was slouched in the corner of a Parisian club, a vague blueprint of the girl I thought I knew. She scowled in my direction. The same pouty expression that was so charming on MySpace was terrifying in real life. She looked different from her photos—not glamorous; just mean.

We were introduced, and Miss X looked carefully at my face.

"I think I've seen you somewhere before," she said.

I looked carefully back at her. And ironically, despite the hours I had spent studying the cyber-contours of her face, I never would have recognized her.

meredith maran

THE BEAUTIFUL GIRL AND ME

There's a photograph of the two of us in a magazine. The headline: "Beautiful Girl." *The subhead:* "What can a feminist aunt learn from her supermodel niece?"

The girl in question, the beautiful one, is my niece, Josie. She's twenty-three. The fifty-year-old with her arms wrapped around her (twice, it seems) is me. Actually, it *was* me when the photo was taken—six years, fourteen gray hairs, fourteen thousand other age-related indignities, and one big insight ago.

I look at my face in the picture, taking it from the top: a tangled mass of near-black curls, shot through with interstitial strands of white. A forehead the color of clay, cross-hatched with furrows plowed into place by twenty mule teams of worry, draught horses of laughter, oxen straining against the sweat-stained harnesses of time. My grandma Sophie's gracefully arched eyebrows—hers hand-plucked, I realize in retrospect; mine, electrolysis-enhanced. Deep-set, almond-shaped, chestnut-brown eyes reflecting pools of changing weather, bracketed by grooves left behind by the sun. A patrician nose that gives no family secrets away; a loose mauve mouth that doesn't take well to lipstick, to penises, or to the Right Thing to Say. Oval face, pointy chin. That's me.

Snuggled up to me is Josie, whom I've adored since she was five minutes old—the Guess Girl at age twenty, the Maybelline Girl at twenty-one, the beautiful girl all her life. Expertly tousled, wavy hair that's been streaked, dyed, hot-combed, curling-ironed, conked, kinked, sprayed, and gelled so many times by so many stylists for so many cover shoots, its once baby-soft brown crown has become a stiff stranger to my touch. *(Josie, I remember bringing my trembling lips to your newborn head, the beat of your brand-new heart visible in those impossibly fragile fontanels, matted in downy dark fuzz.)* A forehead the color of clay, smooth and innocent, a virgin field untrampled by the pounding jackboots of suffering, of fear, of time.

Her great-grandmother Sophie's gracefully arched eyebrows, now professionally tended by the Best in the Biz. Wide, almond-shaped, yellow-specked brown eyes—sun-splashed lakes lit from below by joy and confidence and true grit. A long, straight nose that keeps the family secret; a full, rosy mouth that has made millions by making millions of girls want whatever color was painted upon it—Maybe she's born with it; maybe it's Maybelline—but that speaks its piece, takes no guff, gives as good as it gets. Gives better. Oval face, pointy chin. That's Josie.

The photo was taken to accompany an interview I did with Josie, a public version of the private conversation ("argument," I called it; "my aunt staying on my case," she called it) that she and I have been having since she started modeling at age twelve.

(Josie, I remember your grinning out at me from the Macy's sale insert in my very own Sunday paper. And then pursing your maybe-she's-born-with-it glossy lips at me from a huge display in a Paris grand magasin; staring out at me over your cleavage from store windows on Fifth Avenue; looming nearly naked over Wilshire Boulevard on bigger-than-life Beverly Hills billboards; smiling seductively, your bikini body draped languorously over tropical rocks in the Sports Illustrated swimsuit issue.)

I'd pitched the interview idea to a women's magazine I often wrote for, a magazine in which Josie often appeared. They went for it big-time: flew me to L.A. to do the interview and, months later, for a top-of-the-line photo shoot; sent a limo to pick me up at the airport, funded a $200-dollar sushi lunch that Josie and I ate (yes, the size 0 supermodel eats) on her lushly landscaped Malibu Canyon deck, the tape recorder whirring between us.

"When I was your age," I began with characteristic tact, "I was doing useful things. Picketing the Miss America pageant. Writing diatribes against sexism. Growing out my armpit hair. How could you have turned out this way?"

"You get to be creative with your work," Josie said patiently, doing an impressive impersonation of a person who hadn't had this conversation a hundred times before. "I get to be creative with mine."

"But doesn't it bother you," I pressed on, "to be reinforcing a standard of beauty that 99 percent of women can't meet?"

Josie smiled. "I've never believed that you have to look like Barbie to be happy."

"Easy for you to say, Size Zero," I muttered, swallowing my fifth piece of unagi to Josie's one, but who was counting?

"This beauty thing is crazy," Josie said then, suddenly serious. "People look at me, and all they can think about is that I'm pretty. And all I'm thinking is, that's not it."

That's not it, I told myself at the photo shoot three months later, when the wardrobe stylist wheeled in two racks of borrowed next-season designer clothes: size 0 Stella McCartney for Josie, size 10 Prada for me. *That's not it*, I told myself as Josie and I slithered into and out of cashmere and silk, leather and lace, giggling and preening (Josie); stunned anew by the differences in our skin, shapes, sizes (me). Each time I stuffed myself into another outfit, Josie told me how great I looked. Even in my capacity as aunt and builder of self-esteem, somehow I didn't feel the need to return the compliment.

When the magazine came out, I got a call from my agent. "Wow," she said, "you're brave."

Knowing that "brave" is often agent-speak for "You just screwed up your career," I pondered this for a moment.

"Brave because I asked Josie hard questions in a national magazine?" I responded finally. "She's the brave one. She answered them."

"Brave to have had your picture taken with her," my agent explained.

"She's my niece," I said. "I've been having my picture taken with her for twenty-three years."

What followed was what is commonly referred to as a

pregnant pause, which is agent-speak for "This is going to hurt. Don't make me spell it out for you." And then I realized what she was trying to say.

"Don't stand next to the pretty girl," the teen magazines of my girlhood had warned—a prefeminism cardinal rule I'd scorned and ignored when I was ten years old. But now I'd broken it at age fifty, in the pages of a national magazine, no less.

I looked at the picture again. This time I didn't see a sweet, if stylized, image of my beloved niece and me cuddling on her wall-to-wall couch, our hair and makeup done by a team of Hollywood stylists, wearing ten thousand dollars' worth of really nice clothes. I saw an aging woman with a youthful gleam in her eye and a middle-aged thickening on her thighs, enveloping a plump-breasted, rail-thin young woman in her over-enthusiastic, slightly flabby arms. I saw beautiful Josie, and not-so-beautiful me.

The feeling that bubbled up in me had a color, and it was green. For the first time, I questioned the true source of my righteous critique of Josie's career. Was it born of the feminist consciousness I avowed—or was it proof that jealousy is just as powerful as sisterhood? I'd spent years begging Josie to stop participating in the brainwashing of impressionable young girls. Now I realized that the fire that lit my fervor was the impression that that very brainwashing had made on me.

Six years later, our whole family flies to L.A. to celebrate the first birthday of Josie's beautiful daughter, Rumi Joon. We troop to Rumi's party in the bougainvillea-draped back yard of Josie's best friend, a fellow mom and fellow size 0 model. We hang out at sidewalk cafés, passing Rumi from knee to knee, watching the leggy starlets strut by. We feed Rumi sand-specked strawberries at the beach, while around us, legions of bikini babes frolic cellulitelessly.

Damn digital camera: I come home with 240 photographs. I load them into my iPhoto library to try and cull a few. And then, like a lovestruck teenager, I sit there mesmerized; I click, I coo. *Awww, there's Rumi blowing out the single candle on her vegan birthday cake. Ooh, Rumi gumming a bagel. Ha, Rumi eating chubby handfuls of sand at Zuma Beach.* One photo shows the four generations of women our family now contains: my eighty-year-old mother, fifty-five-year-old me, twenty-nine-year-old Josie, one-year-old Rumi Joon.

Wait. I fill the screen with the photo and sit and stare. I notice that if I compare my face with my mother's, I look like a teenager. When I compare my face with Josie's, I look like a crone. I notice that compared with Rumi's, even Josie's face bears some evidence of having lived a few years on this earth.

I click on to the next image. Josie and I are hugging each other, laughing into each other's eyes. I notice something new. More than wrinkles and age spots have been added to the picture. Our relationship has changed. Josie's a woman now, a mother, a model, and, yes, an entrepreneur. The girl I harangued about doing something "useful" with her life is launching a line of organic cosmetics, hoping to raise money for environmental education in schools.

I'm not just Josie's nagging, do-gooder aunt anymore. I'm the one she calls to edit her website, rewrite her press releases, screen the nonprofits she's considering as partners. Josie's not just my supermodel niece anymore. She's a young woman I mentor. She's a young woman I admire.

If I look from my face to Josie's in order to measure smoothness of skin, symmetry of features, I see only that: flesh covering bone, the flukes of geometry. If I search our faces for what's in our hearts—if I take pride in being Josie's pain-in-the-ass aunt, her editor, her elder, with all the benefits to both of us that those roles entail—I find a lasting beauty, the kind that transcends even time.

alix kates shulman
NOT BAD

I'm seventy-five. Yet when I look in the mirror, the face I see is the same old pal of a face I've had since puberty. Same deep-set green eyes, fine brown hair, arched eyebrows, small nose, full mouth, straightened teeth, Tartar cheekbones. Having regarded it every day of my life, I don't notice the changes. Older, of course, I know, and lined, but not unpleasantly so, not remarkably so, not even (to me) noticeably so. In fact, my face may now be my favorite body part. It wasn't always; in my youth it caused me no end of distress, because I didn't know how it looked to others and couldn't bear the uncertainty. Now I see a face almost generic in its lack of distinction, except, perhaps, for the glint in my eye when I kick up my heels.

I recognize that my sense of it as generic is an illusion, perhaps born of familiarity. But in the mirror, what isn't illusion?

For instance, in the mirror, I see myself only in repose. The strong emotions, which abound in life, are seldom expressed into a mirror. This is probably the reason that Jews in mourning are commanded to cover up all the mirrors in the house—to hide from themselves the ravages of grief. Once, when I was a young mother, my momentary anger at my child so distorted my face that he looked at me in amazement and asked, "Mommy? Is that you?" But when I regard myself in the mirror, I peer out of my face as placidly as a dog peers out of hers.

I know that my view of my face as essentially unchanged isn't widely shared. Away from the mirror, even I acknowledge the more conventional view by rushing to say my name whenever I run into people I haven't seen in ages, in order to save them the embarrassment of not recognizing me. And yes, I'm fussy about my photographs and am reluctant to have a fresh photo taken for the jacket of my next book, preferring the mirror, with all its ambiguity and illusion, to the camera (though frankly, no jacket photo has ever pleased me—a dissatisfaction I attribute to the disparity between my actual face and the one my vanity delivers).

To see myself through others' eyes takes struggle. Only if I exert myself can I make out in the mirror my deeply sunken eyes, gray hairs, thinning eyebrows, puckered mouth, discolored teeth, hollow cheeks, fuzzy jawline. . . . But why bother when there's nothing to be done about it? (Forget makeup, which I've always avoided—not out of aloofness or purity, but rather out of an embarrassed vanity that recoils at such blatant attempts at disguise.) Besides, how is another's view of me any truer, or less tainted, than my own? Even in my youth, when

I was known as a pretty girl, I didn't understand the criteria, didn't get what was meant, though naturally I was grateful for the benefits conferred by other people's inexplicable opinion, as one would be for any piece of good fortune that entail rewards.

Not that I'm blind to those mostly private changes wrought by age—crinkly throat, arms, hands, waist—which I usually conceal discretely beneath long sleeves and high necklines. They sometimes surprise but never baffle me. But when it comes to my face in my forgiving mirror, I see only my dear familiar.

From an early age I was bombarded with warnings that I would inevitably lose my looks and consequent advantages—presumably around the age of thirty. This made me extremely anxious. Anxious to find a less ephemeral, more reliable basis for my place in the world; anxious to secure my future and amount to something before my looks suddenly evaporated, leaving me with nothing. But in those days before feminism (I turned thirty in 1962), my options seemed extremely limited. I was so gripped by our culture's stranglehold on young women's vanity and vulnerability that in the presence of others I was always excruciatingly aware of how I looked—and at the same time uncertain of how I was perceived. Such self-consciousness was almost enough to drive a girl mad.

I might have choked on my own anxiety if feminism hadn't suddenly given me a focus, a purpose, a new idea of growth and expansion to which looks were anything but crucial. Activity in place of passivity. Skill in place of wiles. Self-assertion in place of seduction. Development in place of decay. It enabled me to see women's obsession with looks as an endless trap. In fact, the fledgling women's liberation movement chose the 1968

Miss America pageant in Atlantic City as the site of its splashy national debut: a protest demonstration against oppressive beauty standards, where we (naturally, I was there; wouldn't have missed it) took on a host of hecklers for whom the value of women's beauty was so entrenched that they could interpret our action only as an expression of envy for the contestants.

On that day I lost my concern about losing my looks. Instead, I analyzed the effects of that fear, expressed in my first adult novel, *Memoirs of an Ex-Prom Queen*, which addressed that maddening stranglehold. I saw that my luck was not to have been a pretty girl, but rather to have escaped a pretty girl's fate of forever mourning her lost looks.

Looks, like love, are subjective. Looking at my mate of many years, I find him as beautiful now as when I met him, despite his increasing decrepitude, and can't help but believe his similar declaration when he looks at me, though I realize that he, too, is in the grip of an illusion.

By now my face and I are a smoothly working team, seldom at odds, comfortable together. *Not bad*, I think when I look in the mirror. *Nice smile.*

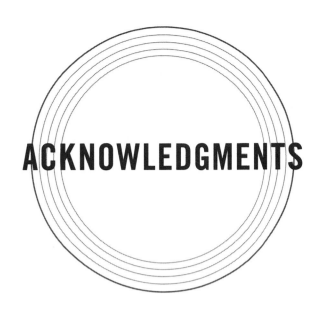

ACKNOWLEDGMENTS

There are as many women behind this book as there are between its covers. We would like to thank, first of all, our contributors, particularly those who were with us from the start and whose insights informed this project: Patricia Chao, Alice Elliott Dark, Susan Davis, Louise DeSalvo, Bonnie Friedman, Meredith Maran, Pamela Redmond Satran, and Kamy Wicoff. We want to thank Catherine Baker, Clara Baker, Cynthia Baker, Gail Belsky, Maureen Connolly, Jess Donohue, Melanie A. Farmer, Naomi Heilig, Gina Hyams, Sheila Kohler, Laura Schenone, Ashley Badger Wakefield, and Bobbi Brown. We also want to thank the women in our Montclair writers' group, whose articulation of their relationships to their own faces, as well as their work as writers, were instrumental in shaping this book.

Our agent, Beth Vesel, has been an enthusiastic advocate and a sounding board from the beginning. Brooke Warner's sharp, incisive editing skills made this collection even stronger.

Seal Press, and particularly its publisher, Krista Lyons-Gould, have always supported our vision for this book. Special thanks to Manijeh Nasrabadi, who worked with us in the early stages as a researcher and editorial assistant, and to the Hunter College Creative Writing Scholarship Program, which funded Manijeh's work with us. Paula Navratil provided much-needed assistance in the later stages. Thanks to the Virginia Center for the Creative Arts for providing the space to contemplate and create the concept for this book. Finally, we want to thank our families—Anne, Craig, Delayna, and Tessa; and Christina, David, Hayden, Will, and Eli—whose patience and unflagging support allowed us to take ourselves away from them long enough to make this book a reality.

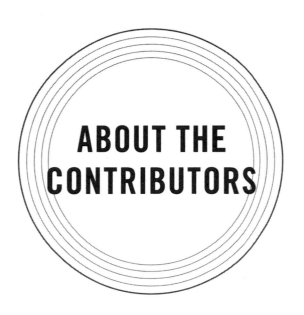

ABOUT THE CONTRIBUTORS

Jennifer Baumgardner is the coauther, with Amy Richards, of two popular Third Wave feminist primers: *Manifesta: Young Women, Feminism, and the Future* and *Grassroots: A Field Guide for Feminist Activism*. She is the producer/creator of the award-winning film *I Had an Abortion* (distributed by Women Make Movies), the controversial T-shirt project of the same name, and a book about women's abortion experiences called *Abortion and Life*. Her book *Look Both Ways: Bisexual Politics* took the pulse of a generation of women increasingly likely to have girlfriends as well as boyfriends. She is currently working on a project about rape.

Bobbi Brown is an internationally renowned make-up artist and CEO of Bobbi Brown Cosmetics. She is the author of *Bobbi Brown Beauty Evolution*, a celebration of beauty across the generations, and coauthor of *Bobbi Brown Beauty* and *Bobbi*

Brown Teenage Beauty. Her products are sold in more than four hundred stores and twenty countries worldwide. In addition to creating cover looks for magazines and making up models for fashion shows, Bobbi is the beauty editor of NBC's *Today Show.* She lives in New Jersey with her husband and three sons.

Kristen Buckley is a screenwriter, novelist, and memoirist. Her credits include *How to Lose a Guy in 10 Days, 102 Dalmatians, The Parker Grey Show,* and *Tramps Like Us.* She is also the cofounder and coeditor of the popular online magazine *The Grange Hall* (www.thregrangehall.com). Prior to her writing career, Buckley worked as a book scout for producer Scott Rudin and as a development executive for Fox 2000.

Marina Budhos is an author of fiction and nonfiction. She has published the novels *Ask Me No Questions, The Professor of Light,* and *House of Waiting* and a nonfiction book, *Remix: Conversations with Immigrant Teenagers.* Her short stories, articles, essays, and book reviews have appeared in publications such as *The Kenyon Review, The Nation, Ms., Travel & Leisure, Time Out,* and the *Los Angeles Times.* She has been a Fulbright scholar to India and received an EMMA (Exceptional Merit Media Award), a Rona Jaffe Award for Women Writers, and a fellowship from the New Jersey Council on the Arts. She is currently on the faculty of the English department at William Paterson University.

Patricia Chao's first novel, *Monkey King,* was a Barnes & Noble Discover Great New Writers finalist. Her second novel, *Mambo*

Peligroso, was derived from her experience as a Latin dancer in New York City. She was awarded a New York Foundation for the Arts fellowship, and her poetry and essays have been published in various journals. She lives in New York City.

Alice Elliott Dark is the author of one novel, *Think of England,* and two collections of short stories, *Naked to the Waist* and *In the Gloaming.* The title story of the latter collection was included in *Best American Stories of the Century,* edited by John Updike, and made into an HBO movie starring Glenn Close and directed by Christopher Reeve. She is working on a new novel called *The Poor Relation.*

Susan Davis is the senior producer of *The State of Things* on North Carolina Public Radio/WUNC. She's the author of a collection of poetry called *Gathering Sound.* She has produced and edited *All Things Considered, Talk of the Nation,* and the National Desk at National Public Radio. Her poems and essays have been heard on many national radio programs and read in many literary journals. She is the coeditor, with Gina Hyams, of the anthology *Searching for Mary Poppins: Women Write About the Intense Relationship Between Mothers and Nannies.* She lives in Chapel Hill, North Carolina, with her husband and two children.

Louise DeSalvo teaches at Hunter College, where she is the Jenny Hunter Endowed Scholar in literature and creative writing. Among other works, she has published four memoirs, including the award-winning *Vertigo* and *Crazy in the Kitchen,* as well as *Writing as a Way of Healing*. She has just completed a book about the significance of the act of moving in her life, her family's, and several writers'.

Bonnie Friedman is the author of the *Village Voice* bestseller *Writing Past Dark: Envy, Fear, Distraction, and Other Dilemmas in the Writer's Life* and *The Thief of Happiness: The Story of an Extraordinary Psychotherapy*. Her essays have appeared in *The Best American Movie Writing, The Best Writing on Writing, The Best Spiritual Writing*, and *O* magazine. She teaches creative nonfiction writing at New York University.

Kathryn Harrison is the author of the novels *Envy, The Seal Wife, The Binding Chair, Poison, Exposure*, and *Thicker Than Water*. Her nonfiction includes the memoirs *The Kiss, The Mother Knot*, and *The Road to Santiago*; a biography, *Saint Thérèse of Lisieux*; a collection of personal essays, *Seeking Rapture*; and a work of true crime, *While They Slept: An Inquiry into the Murder of a Family*. She is a regular reviewer for *The New York Times Book Review*, and her personal essays have appeared in *The New Yorker, Harper's, Vogue, More, O* magazine, and many other publications. She lives in Brooklyn with her husband, the novelist Colin Harrison, and their three children.

Annaliese Jakimides is a writer and visual artist. Her prose and poetry have been published in many journals and magazines, including the *Utne Reader, GQ, Hip Mama, Bangor Metro*, and *Beloit Poetry Journal*, and in collections, most recently *The Long Meanwhile* and *A Seaside Companion*. Her work was broadcast as part of National Public Radio's *This I Believe* series, and she is the editor of the monograph series of Haystack Mountain School of Crafts. A native of Dorchester, Massachusetts, after living for twenty-seven years on forty acres off a dirt road in northern Maine, she now lives in an apartment in the old high school in Bangor, Maine.

Dana Kinstler won the Southern Indiana Review Fiction Prize and the Missouri Review Editors' Prize and has been published in the *Salamander Review* and the *Mississippi Review*. Her essays have appeared or are forthcoming in *Stella* magazine; the *Sunday Telegraph*; *My Father Married Your Mother: Writers Talk about Stepparents, Stepchildren, and Everyone In Between*; *Mr. Wrong*; and *Feed Me*. Her residencies include the Vermont Studio Center and Dorset Colony House. She lives in the Hudson River Valley, New York.

Benilde Little is the author of four best-selling novels: *Good Hair, The Itch, Acting Out,* and *Who Does She Think She Is?* *Good Hair,* which spent six months on the *Essence* bestseller list, was nominated for an NAACP Image Award and named by the *Los Angeles Times* as one of the ten best books of the year. *The Itch* was lauded by Salon.com as a best beach read in the summer of 1998. *Acting Out* won praise in the pages of *Essence, Ebony, The Washington Post,* and *The New York Times Book Review. Who Does She Think She Is?* garnered a front-page Arts section feature in *The New York Times* and was called a "must read" by *The Wall St. Journal.* Little lives in Montclair, New Jersey, with her husband, Clifford, and their two children.

Meredith Maran is the best-selling author of nine books of non-fiction. She is also an award-winning journalist who writes for magazines such as *Salon, Playboy, Self, Family Circle, More,* and *Health.* She's writing her first novel, *A Theory of Small Earthquakes,* about a bisexual with a beautiful face and a troubled soul. You can find her website at www.meredithmaran.com.

Manijeh Nasrabadi graduated from Brown University and received an MFA in creative nonfiction from Hunter College. She is a 2008 recipient of a Hedgebrook Writing Residency and is currently working on a memoir about becoming a part of her extended family in Iran. Queens, New York, and her uncle's house in Tehran are where she feels at home. She can be contacted at manijeh_nasrabadi@yahoo.com.

Ellen Papazian is a Connecticut native who lives in New Jersey with her husband, Kenneth MacBain, and son, Calum River. Her nonfiction work has appeared in *Ms.* and *Hip Mama* magazines. Her short fiction appears in the anthology *The Long Meanwhile: Stories of Arrival and Departure.* She holds a master's degree in English from Rutgers University and just completed her first young-adult novel. Visit her online at www.ellenpapazian.com.

Kym Ragusa is the author of *The Skin Between Us: A Memoir of Race, Beauty, and Belonging,* a finalist for the Hurston/Wright Foundation's 2007 Legacy Award in Nonfiction. She is the recipient of a fellowship from the New York Foundation for the Arts and an Ida and Daniel Lang Award for excellence in the humanities. Her films, *Passing* and *Fuori/Outside,* have been shown on PBS and at festivals throughout North America and Europe. She teaches nonfiction writing in the MFA program at Queens University in Charlotte, North Carolina.

Jade Sanchez-Ventura is a writer of narrative nonfiction. She recently completed her MFA at Hunter College and is working on her first memoir, a tale of a mixed-raced identity, a bohemian upbringing, a snowball incident, Mexico, New York, the Ivy League on scholarship, and the roads between. She lives in Brooklyn.

Pamela Redmond Satran is the author of four novels—*Suburbanistas, Younger, Babes in Captivity,* and *The Man I Should Have Married*—and coauthor of eight best-selling baby-naming guides, including *The Baby Name Bible* and *Cool Names for Babies.* A columnist for *Glamour* and a blogger for *The Huffington Post,* Satran has written essays and articles for publications ranging from *The New York Times* to *Parenting* to *Publisher's Weekly* and *Bon Appétit.* She and her husband—Richard Satran, an editor at Reuters—have three children.

Rory Satran was born in New York in 1982 and studied comparative literature at the University of California, Berkeley. In 2002 she moved to Paris, where she became a freelance writer for such publications as *The Washington Post* and *Marie Claire.* Since 2006, Satran has been the managing editor of the fashion and culture biannual magazine *Self Service.* Her literary work is represented by the Irene Goodman Agency in New York.

Alix Kates Shulman is the author of twelve books, including novels, memoirs, a biography, and children's books. A thirty-fifth-anniversary edition of her first novel, the feminist classic *Memoirs of an Ex-Prom Queen*, was issued in 2007. Her newest book, *To Love What Is*, delves into the terrors and rewards of caring for a beloved, brain-injured husband. Long a committed social activist, organizer, and teacher, she has taught widely in U.S. universities and has received numerous awards, including an honorary doctorate from Case Western Reserve University in 2001.

Catherine Texier grew up and was educated in France, and she writes both in French and in English. She is the author of four novels—*Victorine*, *Chloé l'Atlantique*, *Love Me Tender*, and *Panic Blood*—and a memoir, *Breakup*. She was coeditor, with Joel Rose, of the literary magazine *Between C & D*, and is the recipient of a National Endowment for the Arts Award and two New York Foundation for the Arts fellowships. She teaches creative writing at the New School and at Brooklyn College. She has lived in Paris and Montreal and now lives in New York City.

S. Kirk Walsh's essays have appeared in *My Father Married Your Mother* and *Pissed Off: On Women and Anger*. She writes book reviews for *The New York Times* and is a frequent contributor to *T: The New York Times Magazine*. Her awarded residencies include the Ragdale Foundation and the Virginia Center for the Creative Arts. Currently, Walsh is completing a novel. She lives in Austin, Texas, and is a founding board member of Austin Bat Cave, a writing center for kids.

Kamy Wicoff is the author of the best-selling book *I Do But I Don't: Why the Way We Marry Matters*. Her work has appeared in Salon.com, *Redbook*, and *WSQ* and in the anthology *Why I'm Still Married: Women Write Their Hearts Out on Love, Loss, Sex, and Who Does the Dishes*. She and her husband, Andrew, live in New York City with their sons, Maximilian and Jedidiah.

ABOUT THE EDITORS

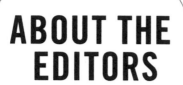

Anne Burt is the editor of *My Father Married Your Mother: Dispatches from the Blended Family.* In addition to being widely anthologized, her essays have appeared in publications including *Real Simple,* Salon.com, *Working Mother, Parenting,* and *The Christian Science Monitor* and on National Public Radio's *All Things Considered* and *Talk of the Nation.* Burt has appeared on *The Today Show* and *ABC News Now* to speak about stepparenting, and writes a monthly column, "Musings from the Evil Stepmother," for DivineCaroline.com. She won *Meridian* literary magazine's 2002 Editors' Prize in Fiction and is at work on a novel. Burt lives in New Jersey with her husband, daughter, and stepdaughter and works at Columbia University.

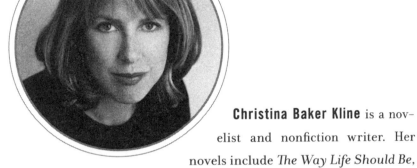

Christina Baker Kline is a novelist and nonfiction writer. Her novels include *The Way Life Should Be*, *Desire Lines*, and *Sweet Water*. She is coauthor, with Christina L. Baker, of *The Conversation Begins: Mothers and Daughters Talk About Living Feminism*, and editor of *Child of Mine, Room to Grow*, and *Always Too Soon*. Currently writer in residence at Fordham University, Kline has also taught literature and creative writing at Yale, NYU, the University of Virginia, and Drew University. She is a graduate of Yale, Cambridge University, and the University of Virginia, where she was a Henry Hoyns Fellow in Fiction Writing. She is a 2007 recipient of a Geraldine R. Dodge Foundation fellowship at the Virginia Center for the Creative Arts.

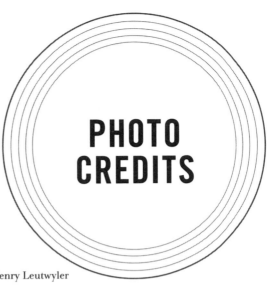

PHOTO CREDITS

Selected Titles from Seal Press

For more than thirty years, Seal Press has published ground-breaking books. By women. For women. Visit our website at www.sealpress.com.

bOObs: A Guide to Your Girls by Elisabeth Squires. $15.95, 1-58005-207-X. Funny and thoroughly thought-provoking, this useful owner's manual will improve every woman's relationship with her breasts.

For Keeps: Women Tell the Truth About Their Bodies, Growing Older, and Acceptance edited by Victoria Zackheim. $15.95, 1-58005-204-5. This inspirational collection of personal essays explores the relationship that aging women have with their bodies.

It's So You: 35 Women Write About Personal Expression Through Fashion and Style edited by Michelle Tea. $15.95, 1-58005-215-0. From the haute couture houses of the ruling class to DIY girls who make restorative clothing and create their own hodgepodge style, this is the first book to explore women's ambivalence toward, suspicion of, indulgence in, and love of fashion on every level.

The Bigger, The Better, The Tighter the Sweater edited by Samantha Schoech and Lisa Taggart. $14.95, 1-58005-210-X. A refreshingly honest and funny collection of essays on how women view their bodies.

Kill the Princess: Why Women Still Aren't Free from the Quest for a Fairytale Life by Stephanie Vermeulen. $15.95, 1-58005-223-1. Tackling issues that modern women face, from body image to juggling career and family, this is an in-your-face, empowering wake-up call for women everywhere.

Women in Overdrive: Find Balance and Overcome Burnout at Any Age by Nora Isaacs. $14.95, 1-58005-161-8. For women who take on more than they can handle, this book highlights how women of different age sets are affected by overdrive, and what they can do to avoid burnout.